Yoga Posture Adjustments and Assisting

An Insightful Guide for Yoga Teachers and Students

BY STEPHANIE PAPPAS
DIRECTOR OF DEVALILA YOGA TEACHER TRAINING

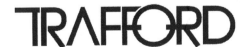

Note for Librarians: A cataloguing record for this book is available from Library and Archives Canada at www.collectionscanada.ca/amicus/index-e.html
ISBN 1-4120-5162-2

Photographic models (photos used with permission): Stephanie Pappas, Carla Robert, Dawn Sharp, Carrie Colditz, Heidi Prewett, Elizabeth Gill, John Feddersen, Martha Watson, Linda Wellbrock (all certified Devalila Yoga teachers!)

Book photographs by: Stephanie Pappas, Manuel Cano Diaz, and the photographic models

Author: Stephanie Pappas (a.k.a. Stefani Pappas)

Editors: Valery Keith, June Pettinelly

Book cover design: Stephanie Pappas and Trafford Publishing designers

Book interior design: Stephanie Pappas

Design consultants: Dori Urquhardt, Kirk Bobash, Jennifer Dedrick

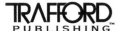

Offices in Canada, USA, Ireland and UK

This book was published *on-demand* in cooperation with Trafford Publishing. On-demand publishing is a unique process and service of making a book available for retail sale to the public taking advantage of on-demand manufacturing and Internet marketing. On-demand publishing includes promotions, retail sales, manufacturing, order fulfilment, accounting and collecting royalties on behalf of the author.

Book sales for North America and international:
Trafford Publishing, 6E–2333 Government St.,
Victoria, BC V8T 4P4 CANADA
phone 250 383 6864 (toll-free 1 888 232 4444)
fax 250 383 6804; email to orders@trafford.com
Book sales in Europe:
Trafford Publishing (UK) Limited, 9 Park End Street, 2nd Floor
Oxford, UK OXI IHH UNITED KINGDOM
phone 44 (0)1865 722 113 (local rate 0845 230 9601)
facsimile 44 (0)1865 722 868; info.uk@trafford.com
Order online at:
trafford.com/05-0057

10   9   8   7   6   5   4   3

DEDICATION

જ જ જ

I would like to dedicate this book to all the yoga teachers who have graduated from the Devalila Yoga Teacher Training and other trainings I have given, and all the yoga and belly dance students who have attended my classes throughout the years. It is because of your openness, willingness, and receptivity that I have been able to share my experience of yoga, dance, and life, and in turn, learn so much from you all. I would also like to express my gratitude to my formal teachers of yoga, meditation and Buddhism: Sri Sri Ravi Shankar, His Holiness the 14th Dalai Lama, Osho, Pema Chödrön, Kirin Mishra and Bobbie Ellis. A special thanks to Manuel Cano Diaz, my family, my friends Dori and Kirk, and the Devalila teacher graduates of 2004 for giving me the camera to make this book: John Feist, Jim Johnston, Carrie Colditz, Whitney Frith, Melissa Stern, Elizabeth Gill, and Katherine Doyle.

Contents

"Things are as bad, and as good as they seem—there's no need to add anything extra."
—Buddha

Section I

Introduction to Yoga Posture Adjustments and Assisting

Getting Started

Whether you are a new or experienced yoga teacher or student, you can reap the benefits of learning to give and receive yoga posture adjustments.

Receiving assistance in a yoga posture can be a wonderful experience. When my teacher first assisted me, I felt as if I were getting a great massage while doing my yoga practice. It was like a dream come true! Over time I experienced a big improvement in my range of motion and ability to relax in the postures. I was able to balance better and stretch much further after being assisted. Later when I practiced on my own, my body remembered where it had gone with the help of the teacher, and I went much deeper into the postures. In addition to the physical benefits, I felt nurtured, acknowledged, and grateful for the extra attention.

In this introductory section I explain the foundations of posture adjusting. This section should prepare you to perform the actual techniques in the second section. After reading the introductory section you can skip to any chapter in Section II containing the postures you want to work on.

In the third section I offer my replies to questions from yoga teachers and students that I have received over the years. I hope you find it thought provoking and refreshing.

The most important points to remember when using this book are:

- Use caution and compassion when working with someone else's body. Everyone's body is unique. You don't need to exactly mimic the photos.

- Move slowly, carefully, and consciously when adjusting someone.

- Ask for feedback and heed your partner's requests to stop or release the adjustments. Never force someone into a posture.

So, get out your yoga mat and props, put on some music, and have fun exploring the yoga postures in a whole new way!

Language and Terms Used in this Book

In order to teach yoga posture adjustments to yoga teachers in training, I use some unique terms to describe the subtle movements and unusual body positions that are used. Review these terms before performing the techniques presented in Section II:

Assisting/Assist/Assistance

I define assisting, an assist, or giving assistance as the act of physically stretching, pressing, moving or touching someone while they are in a yoga posture. By my definition, assisting lasts a longer than an adjustment, and uses a deeper pressure. The aim of assisting is to take someone deeper in the pose, correct postural misalignments, and encourage exploration and greater movement.

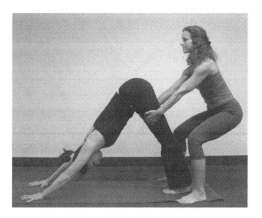

Adjusting

I define adjusting as the act of making a simple, short alteration or correction to a yoga posture. By my definition, adjusting is of a shorter duration than assisting and utilizes a lighter touch. The aim of adjusting is to encourage a small movement, a subtle awareness, a change in position, or a relaxation of a certain part of the body. The photos below show an adjustment of knee position in a warrior two pose.

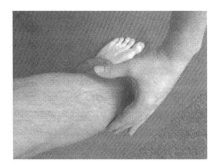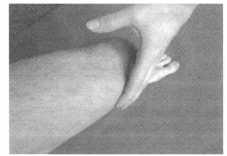

The "Catcher's" Position

The "catcher's" position gives you leverage and stability when assisting people who are on the floor doing forward bending, twisting, and folding type postures. It looks like the position that some baseball catchers use at home base. It is a half squat position with one knee or the whole shin touching the floor. Your back foot can be positioned on the ball of the foot (left photo), or the top of the foot (right photo).

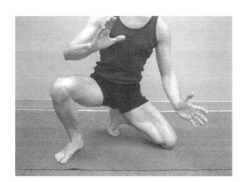 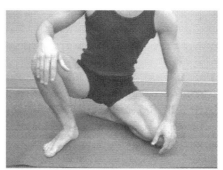

The "Marriage Proposal" Position

The "marriage proposal" position gives you stability when assisting people who are on the floor or standing in postures. It looks like the old-fashioned position for proposing marriage. In this position, one knee is on the floor and one knee is bent at a right angle. Your back foot can be positioned on the ball of the foot or the top of the foot.

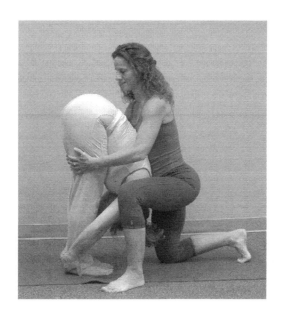

"Opening the Refrigerator"

When you approach your refrigerator to get something you approach it head on with your hand naturally reaching out for the handle, right? Well, when you approach someone to assist or adjust, keep in mind the notion of opening your refrigerator. Your alignment and body mechanics are just as important as the person you are assisting.

When people begin to practice assisting their tendency is to approach the person being assisted at an awkward angle, and usually from a position too far away from the body of the student. An unbalanced approach can create strain in your body and also make the assistance ineffective. Remember to approach the person in a direct fashion, keep your spine lengthened, and to apply pressure using your body weight. If you feel you are working hard, chances are you are using too much of your muscle strength and not enough leverage. The assistant on the left is using better body mechanics than the assistant on the right.

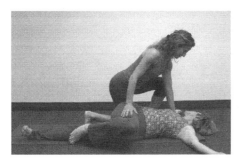 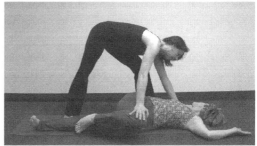

"Grounded" Stance

In a "grounded" stance your legs are wide apart, your feet are flat, and your knees are bent. A grounded stance feels stable and strong, and has a sense of balance. This stance is essential when assisting someone in a standing or balancing posture. The stance on the left below is more stable than the stance on the right.

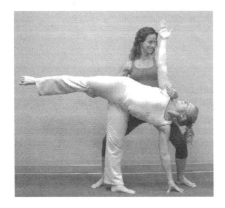 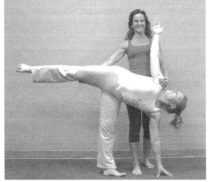

No "Pokey" Hands

I use the word "pokey" to describe the way a person's fingers can feel on your body when they are using just the tips of their fingers instead of their whole hand. A pokey adjustment can feel like you are being prodded instead of touched. Remember to use your whole hand and have the intention of making solid contact with the body of your student. In the photo on the left the assistant is using a firm contact.

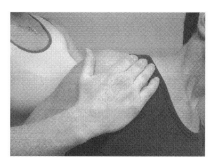 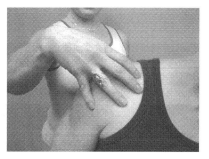

The "Edge"

I refer to the "edge" as that time and place in the posture when you feel just enough sensation, but not too much. When you reach your edge, you should still be able to breathe deeply. Even though you are at your edge, you are not straining your body in the position, and the sensation you feel is somewhere between comfort and moderate discomfort.

The "Mound"

I refer to the "mound" as the area that protrudes around the lower inside edge of the scapula blade when someone is turning their torso and shoulders. The mound is an effective spot to place the heel of your hand when you are assisting someone in a revolving posture.

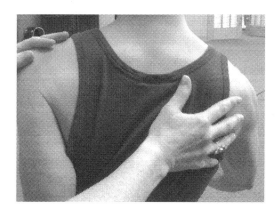

The "Straddle" Position

In the "straddle" position your legs are spread apart and you are standing over a part of the person's body. Straddling someone allows you to have better access to their body and get more leverage. When straddling someone you can assist them with less strain and a straighter spine.

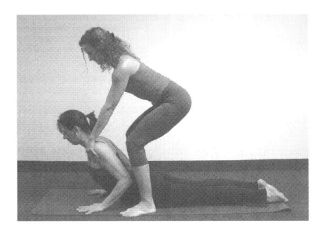

The "Skiers Squeeze" Position

In the "skier's squeeze" position you are standing in a bent knee position with your feet fairly close together (as in chair pose or when you are skiing), and you are actively squeezing a person's leg with your inner thighs or knees. This position is a very effective way to stabilize the base of a standing pose.

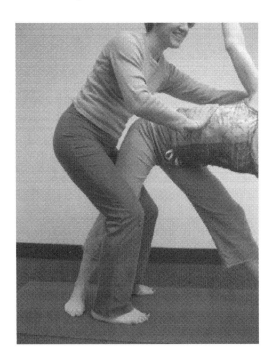

The "Standing Squat" Position or "Horse" Stance

In the "horse" stance or "standing squat" position your legs are spread apart in a wide stance, and your knees are bent and in alignment with your feet. Your spine is erect and your feet are firmly planted on the floor. Your body feels like it is sinking downward toward the earth. Remember to keep your navel drawn in toward your spine. You may need to change the depth of the squat depending on the height of the person and the yoga pose they are performing. Use this stance to remain stable and balanced when you are assisting someone in a standing posture.

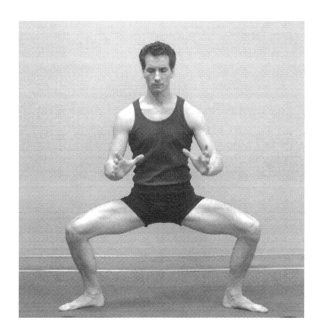

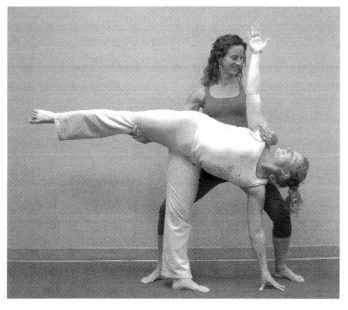

The "High or Low Lunge" Position

Assisting someone from a high or low lunge position gives you leverage and allows you to use your body weight instead of muscle force. In the lunge position you can work with gravity and utilize the strength of your legs to give a balanced, deep pressure. The top photo shows the low lunge position. The bottom photo shows the high lunge position.

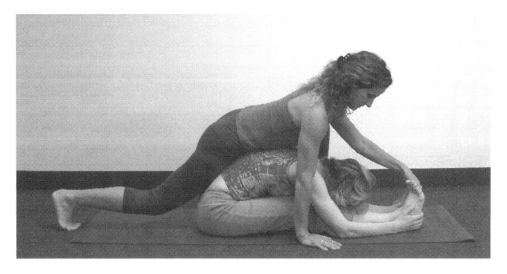

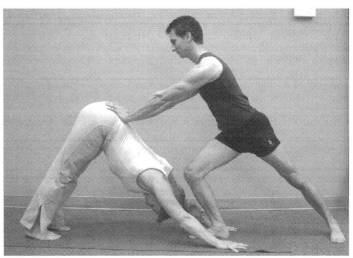

"Opening a Jar"

When you open a jar you need to hold one end tightly while you pry the jar lid open, right? The same principle applies when you are assisting someone in a twisting pose. When you want to twist their torso or shoulders, you must steady the base of their body first (like you would the bottom of a jar), and then twist their torso (like you would the top of a jar). You can provide more support and movement if you apply this principle while assisting.

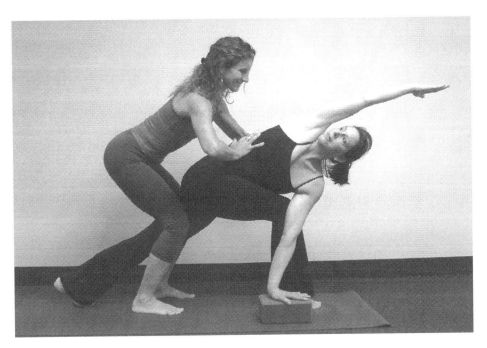

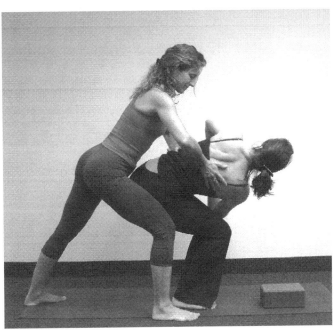

Adjusting and Assisting Tips

Here are some great tips for adjusting and assisting yoga postures in class or in private sessions. Remember that these are tips, not rules, and they may not apply certain situations. The posture adjustment you decide to give will depend on the person's needs and ability, your intuition, and your mood.

Ask Precise Questions

In order to receive specific feedback about your assistance you need to ask specific questions. It is more effective to ask a person if they would like more or less pressure, rather than simply asking them if the pressure is okay. Your verbal interactions can be more extensive in private sessions. In classroom settings you have less time to talk. Honor a student's request even if you want to do something different. The feedback you get will allow you to quickly modify your actions to meet the needs of the person.

Keep Your Attention on the Breath

Listen to their breath while you are assisting. If you can't hear it, watch for it in the movements of their abdomen, sternum, shoulders and upper back. Listen to your own breath as well. Are you breathing? Adjust their posture in harmony with their breath. Sometimes you can encourage them to breathe more deeply by breathing in a slightly audible manner yourself (ujjayi breath). When you assist people in poses that twist or contract (like revolving or folding postures), it's best to apply more pressure on their **exhalation**. When you assist people in poses that expand and lift (like back bends), it's best to apply more pressure on the **inhalation**.

Adjust the Most Unsafe Misalignments First

Don't waste your time adjusting an insignificant part of their body when another part of their body is in a bad position that could cause injury in the short or long term. When you notice that several or many people in class are similarly misaligned, verbally correct them before trying to manually adjust everyone. When you feel it is necessary, have everyone come out of a posture, watch you demonstrate the correct alignment, and then perform the pose a second time.

Stabilize (Ground) Your Body before Assisting Someone

If you start to assist someone with an unstable posture yourself, there is more of a chance that the both of you may feel uneasy, and in certain circumstances you could both fall over. If you are not grounded, you are more likely to strain yourself and less likely to apply a deep, steady pressure.

Apply Pressure in the Correct Direction

Carefully observe the person in the posture and notice the direction in which they are moving (or want to move). Move them in the same direction. This may seem obvious, but in twisting poses there can be confusion.

Walk Away Gradually after Adjusting or Assisting

Make sure that the person in the pose is stable and balanced before you walk away. If you walk away abruptly after a deep assist, they may fall over. I like to leave one of my hands on their lower back as I move away from a standing pose. Sometimes all it takes is leaving one of your fingers in contact with their body to help them remain stable.

Explain Assisting to New Students before the Class Begins

When you start a new class, briefly discuss posture adjustments and assisting. If one or two new students join your ongoing class, explain assisting to them privately before the class begins. By explaining beforehand you can avoid possible confusion and misunderstandings.

Assess an Appropriate Duration for Your Assistance

The duration of your assistance depends greatly on the posture, the situation, and the student. In a classroom setting, you can start by assisting for about 3-5 deep breaths if they are in a basic pose such as cobra or downward dog. In private sessions, you can assist them for several minutes or more. The time you spend also depends on the person's current needs and ability. Give them time to sink into the pose. Don't change your hand positions too quickly. There are times to assist, and not to assist. You will become more intuitive as you practice on people. Keep in mind these questions while assisting someone:

Are they going deeper and relaxing into the posture?
If they are, you may want to stay longer so that they can go even deeper. If they aren't, you may want to leave them alone. If you feel stiffness, resistance, or notice that their breath is shallow, encourage them to breathe a little deeper. You can also offer some type of yoga prop to help them relax into the posture.

Is my intention to give a light adjustment or a deep assist?
If your intention is to give a light directional adjustment (such as moving their foot or hand) then you may only need to be with them for a few seconds. If your intention is to give a deeper stretch, then you may need to be with them for a minute or more.

Is this student beginning, intermediate, or advanced?
The ability and needs of a student can vary from day to day, class to class. Sometimes you may want to spend more time with a beginner because they need help, and less time with an advanced student because they are familiar with the practice. At other times you may want to spend more time giving a deep assist to an advanced student, and less time making a short adjustment for a beginner. Your skills will improve as you get to know your students.

Be Conscious of Your Noise Level

Strike a balance between being too quiet and too noisy as you walk around the classroom. Try not to startle the students by approaching them too softly, but also don't walk around creating so much noise that your presence is a distraction. When you are in a private setting, avoid over talking.

Use Soft Verbal Instructions While Assisting in the Classroom

It is helpful to give soft verbal instructions when you are assisting someone so that they more clearly understand what you want them to do. Keep your voice low so that you don't distract the nearby students.

Some teachers ask permission every time they touch someone in class. I feel this is unnecessary and can be annoying to the students. With a new student you may want to ask their permission the first time you touch them, but I think it's it is more effective to discuss this before class begins.

Avoid Overcorrecting

No one likes to feel like they are doing something wrong—especially when they are trying something new. Correction is good, but overcorrecting can leave the student feeling like a failure or frustrated. Be compassionate when adjusting and try to put yourself in their shoes as much as possible.

Be Specific with Your Touch

Be conscious of your hand placement while assisting someone. Avoid accidentally touching sensitive areas (groin, armpits, buttocks, breasts). Remember that some people may have ticklish spots unknown to you. I suggest that you refrain from random touches (petting, patting, stroking) that lack a specific intention to adjust the posture.

Keep Part of Your Attention on the Whole Class While Assisting

When you are assisting one person in a classroom setting, continue to observe the rest of the class and give them verbal instructions. Don't leave the class in the postures too long because you are busy helping one person.

Stay Aware of Your Body Mechanics

Notice when your body is uncomfortable while assisting. Are you hunching over? Lean into the posture and not away from the posture. Use the strength of your feet and legs. The left photo is an example of ineffective body mechanics. The right photo is an example of effective body mechanics.

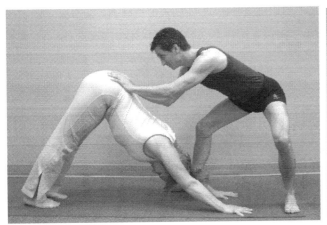 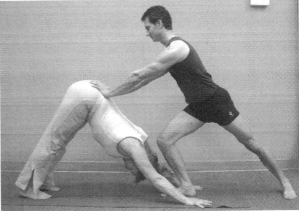

Use Creative Body Positions

There are many ways to use your whole body or parts of your body while assisting. The photos below are examples of body positions involving the back, foot, shin, and ankles. I encourage you to experiment with the techniques in Section II, and you can invent your own positions once you become more familiar and comfortable with assisting.

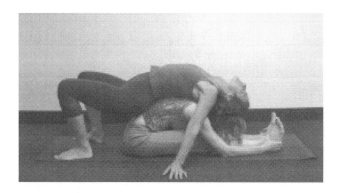

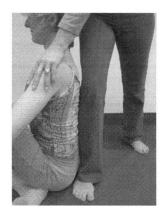

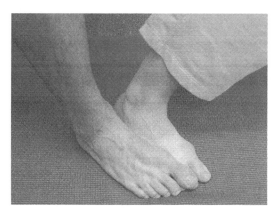

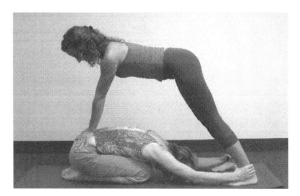

Give Out Props: Blocks, Blankets, Pillows, Chairs and Straps

You can give out many types of props to help your students attain comfort and safety in the postures. Make props available before the start of the yoga pose if possible, or hand them out while the person is performing a pose. It is useful if you have enough props for everyone in the class. You can ask students to bring their own props to class as well. Make sure the props are readily accessible before you start your class or private session. Some ways to use props are demonstrated in the photos below:

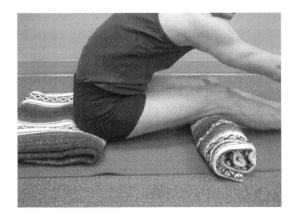
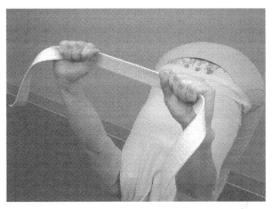

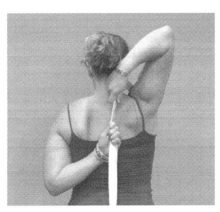
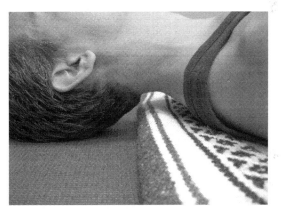

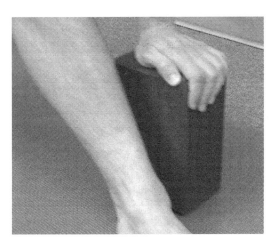

Section II

Posture Adjustments and Assisting

Standing Postures

People generally find the standing poses more physically challenging and may not hold the postures for too long. This means you have less time to set up and apply the techniques. In the standing poses you act as a support and an anchor for the person in the pose. Standing poses can be tricky because of the balance component. Here are some points to remember when assisting someone in the standing poses presented in this chapter:

- Perform standing assists with a solid, grounded stance or you both may become unstable and could fall over. This can bring some laughs, but also some danger.

- Avoid throwing them off balance by coming up to them too close or too quick. With poses like dancer and tree for example, you are only standing an inch or two away from their body, or slightly touching.

- Stabilize the pose first in the legs or hips before taking the person deeper into the opening aspect of the pose.

- Back away slowly—gradually let them find their own balance and take their own weight.

- Leave one of your hands on their hip or sacrum as you back away from them so they don't fall over.

- Don't approach them so quietly that you startle them and they lose their equilibrium.

- Don't walk in front of them if they are focusing their eyes on a fixed point for balance.

Note: All the postures in the following section should be performed for at least 20-30 seconds, but can be held for longer depending on the needs of the student.

Mountain

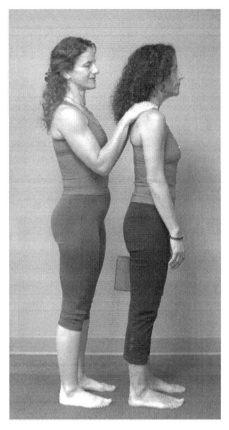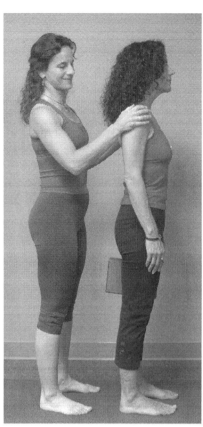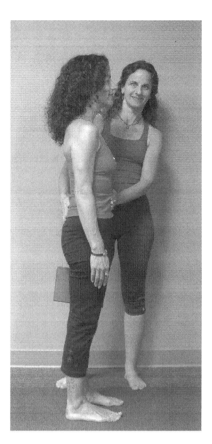

"Take more risks for what you really want in life. Being comfortable does not necessarily bring happiness. Change is usually uncomfortable—it shakes us, and wakes us up. Go for the whole experience of life and open up to different aspects of yourself. Life is a mystery! Maybe there is no resolution." –Stephanie Pappas, Devalila Yoga Teacher and Trainer

Assisting Steps for Mountain Pose

Stand behind the person and place your hands on the top of their shoulders while pressing downward to encourage them to lengthen their neck and relax their shoulders (as in the left photo). You can even give their shoulders a few firm squeezes.

Then, cup your hands around their upper arms (deltoids) and roll them backwards to encourage them to expand their chest (as in the middle photo).

Then, stand to the side of the person and gently press inward around the navel area with one hand, and press downward on the sacrum with the other hand to encourage awareness their pelvic alignment (as in the right photo).

Continue to observe their body in mountain pose and use gentle touch to encourage postural alignment in other areas such as neck, head, rib cage, and feet.

When you are finished, allow them to breath and experience mountain pose.

Yoga Prop Suggestions

Have them squeeze a yoga block between their mid to upper thighs to stabilize and engage the legs.

What You Might Say (to help the process)

"Spread your toes," "Firm the lower abs and bring your navel toward the spine," "Drop your tail bone," "Let your shoulders relax."

> "Being assisted allows me to experience a range of movement I never thought possible. I feel lighter, more spacious…" –Deana Stevens, Psy.D, Devalila Yoga Teacher

Arching Mountain

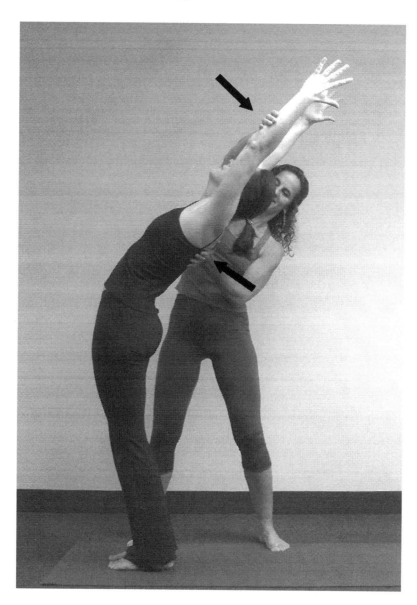

Assisting Steps for Arching Mountain Pose

Stand to one side of the person.

Place your open hand on their back between their shoulder blades and press upward to give a lifting/supportive sensation.

Simultaneously place your other hand and forearm across their arms and press them backwards into a gentle arch.

Deepen the assist on their exhalation.

Release your hands and allow them to return to a normal standing position.

Yoga Prop Suggestions

Have them squeeze a yoga block between their mid to upper thighs to stabilize and engage the legs.

Have them hold a yoga block between their hands to help engage the arms.

What You Might Say (to help the process)

"Breathe deeply into your upper chest," "Keep your neck long," "Tuck under the tail bone," "Let your shoulders drop down away from your ears."

> "Assisting helps the teacher feel the accomplishment of helping his/her student into a successful pose." –Eloise Sicora, Devalila Yoga Teacher, Pilates Teacher

Tree

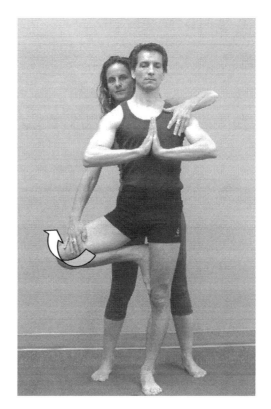

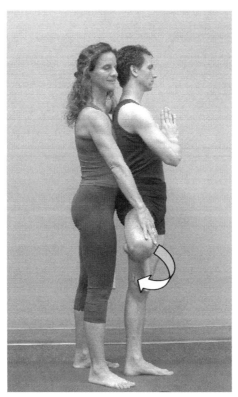

Assisting Steps for Tree Pose

Stand in a grounded stance behind the person almost touching them.

Carefully and slowly, place one hand on their front deltoid. Simultaneously, place your other hand on their inner knee or slightly above the inner knee of the bent leg.

Help them balance in the pose and then slightly draw their shoulder and knee backward to create an opening feeling in the front body and hip.

Allow their back body to touch your chest, ribs or stomach for support as they deepen in the pose.

Maintain the assistance for as long as you feel is appropriate. Stay aware of their body and yours, and listen for their breath.

Release your hands slowly, back away, and allow them to find their equilibrium.

Perform the assist on the other side.

Yoga Prop Suggestions

Have them stand facing a wall, or sideways next to a wall, so they may touch it with their hand for balance.

What You Might Say (to help the process)

"Let your tailbone drop down,", "Press your foot firmly into your inner thigh," "Draw your navel inward," "Keep your hips parallel to the floor."

"Breathe, just breathe and relax. The most extraordinary asana will flow through you and the class."—John Feddersen, Devalila Yoga Teacher

Chair

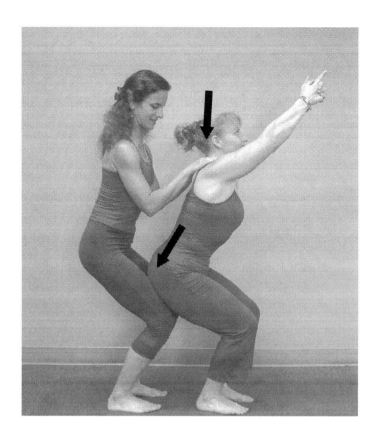

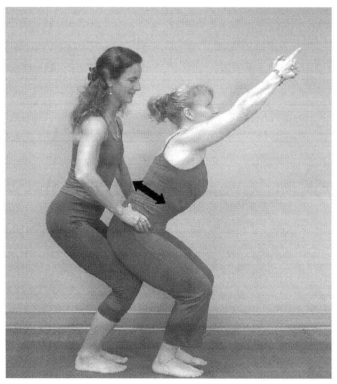

Assisting Steps for Chair Pose

Stand behind the person with slightly bent knees as in chair pose.

Guide their hips to sit onto your thighs and take some of the weight.

Use your free hands to depress their shoulders, draw in the rib cage, or tilt the pelvis to a neutral position. Your action depends on how you perceive their alignment and where you notice they are holding tension.

Maintain the assistance for as long as you feel is appropriate. Stay aware of their body and yours, and listen for their breath.

Release your hands, and allow them to return to mountain position.

Yoga Prop Suggestions

Have them squeeze a yoga block between their knees to stabilize and engage the legs.

Have them hold a yoga block between their hands to help engage the arms.

What You Might Say (to help the process)

"Relax your jaw, face and neck," "Soften your rib cage," "Draw navel inward toward your spine," "Lower back/sacrum finds a neutral position."

"When I was being assisted, I felt more secure and was able to experience the deeper posture without fear of losing my balance or injuring myself."
–Daniel Farrell, Devalila Yoga Teacher, Scientist

Eagle

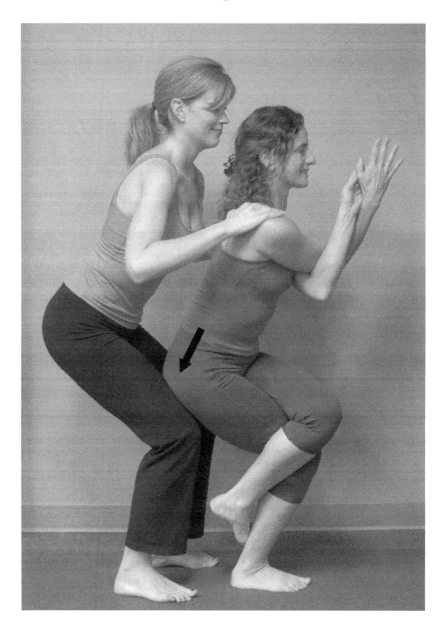

Assisting Steps for Eagle Pose

Stand behind the person with slightly bent knees as in chair pose.

Guide their hips to sit onto your thighs to take some of the weight.

Use your free hands to depress their shoulders, draw in the rib cage, or tilt the pelvis to a neutral position. Your action depends on how you perceive their alignment and where you notice they are holding tension.

Maintain the assistance for as long as you feel is appropriate. Stay aware of their body and yours, and listen for their breath.

Release your hands and allow them to return to a mountain pose.

Perform the assist on the other side.

Yoga Prop Suggestions

If they can't wrap their foot fully around the ankle, have them touch their big toe to the floor or stay in the chair pose leg position.

What You Might Say (to help the process)

"Squeeze your arms together," "Depress your shoulder blades," "Draw navel inward toward your spine," "Activate your inner thighs."

"Respect the decisions of your students and honor that they have their own inner teachers."
-Stephanie Pappas, Devalila Teacher and Trainer

Standing Leg Extension (Front and Side)

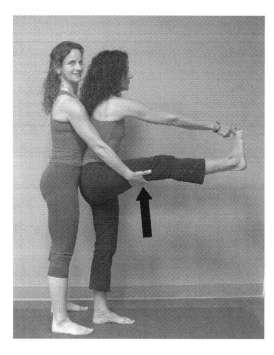

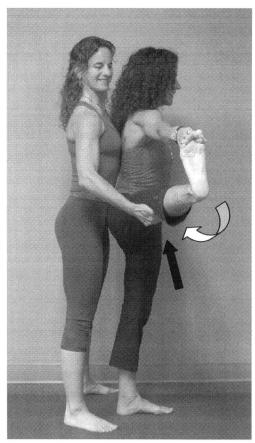

Assisting Steps for Standing Leg Extension Pose

Stand in a grounded stance behind the person almost touching them.

Carefully and slowly, cup one hand around their front upper arm and draw it slightly toward you.

Simultaneously, give support and lift under their outstretched leg (whether it's to the front or to the side) with your other hand.

Allow their back body to touch your chest, ribs or stomach for support as they deepen and balance in the pose.

Maintain the assistance for as long as you feel is appropriate. Stay aware of their body and yours, and listen for their breath.

Release your hands slowly, back away, and allow them to find their balance.

Perform the assist on the other side.

Yoga Prop Suggestions

Have them stand sideways next to a wall so they may touch it for balance with their free hand.

What You Might Say (to help the process)

"Keep your spine upright," "Hold the big toe firmly and lift," "Extend through both legs," "Draw your abdominal muscles firm and drawing inward," "Keep your hips parallel to the floor."

"I just love touching people and being touched. It has always felt very natural to me."
–Stephanie Pappas, Devalila Yoga Teacher and Trainer

Warrior One

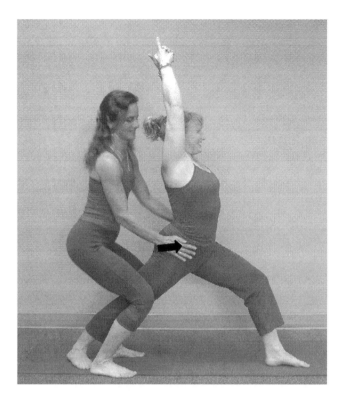

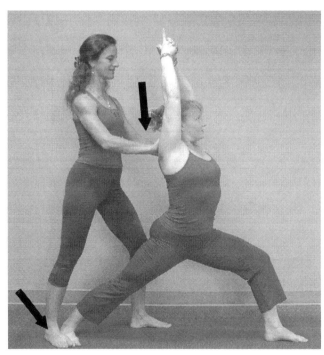

Assisting Steps for Warrior One Pose

Stand behind the person as you anchor their back leg with the skiers squeeze position above their knee area (as in the top photo), or anchor their back foot down with your foot (as in the bottom photo).

Use your free hands to depress their shoulders, draw in the rib cage, or tilt the pelvis to a neutral position. Your action depends on how you perceive their alignment and where you notice they are holding tension.

Maintain the assistance for as long as you feel is appropriate. Stay aware of their body and yours, and listen for their breath.

Release your hands, and allow them to return to mountain position.

Perform the assist on the other side.

Yoga Prop Suggestions

Have them press the outer edge of their back foot against a wall.

Have them hold a yoga block between their hands to help engage the arms.

What You Might Say (to help the process)

"Press both feet fully and firmly into the floor," "Turn your chest toward your front leg," "Drop tail bone down and navel inward," "Let your shoulders relax as you extend your arms."

"As a student, being assisted taught me to let go and accept help."
–Adrienne Yurinko, Devalila Yoga Teacher

Warrior Two—Option 1 Arm Stretch

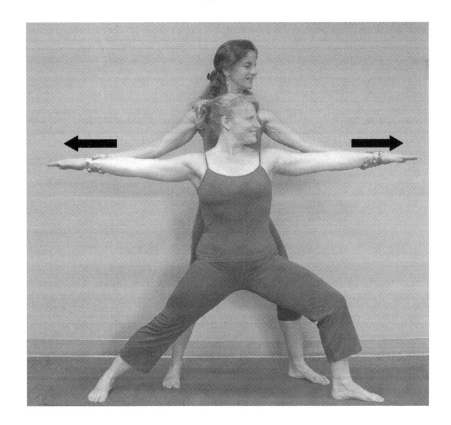

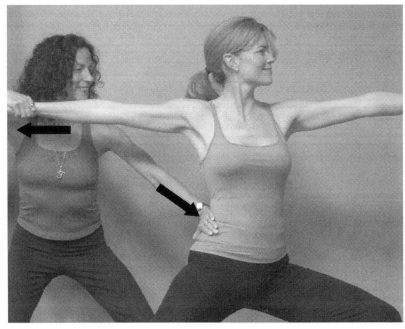

Assisting Steps for Warrior Two Pose (Arm Stretch)

Stand behind the person.

Hold near both their wrists using your thumb and index fingers.

Stretch their arms outward away from their body and maintain traction as they breathe deeply into the upper chest (as in the top photo).

Align their arms in a "T" position and parallel to the floor.

Then, stand near their back leg and pull their back arm toward you while simultaneously pressing into their waist area to bring their torso into alignment with their pelvis (as in the bottom photo).

Maintain the assistance for as long as you feel is appropriate. Stay aware of their body and yours, and listen for their breath.

Release your hands and allow them to return to mountain position, or perform a different assist for warrior two pose.

Perform the assist on the other side.

Yoga Prop Suggestions

Have them press the outer edge of their back foot into a wall.

What You Might Say (to help the process)

"Breath deeply into your upper chest," "Reach out through your fingertips," "Soften the front rib cage," "Let your shoulders relax."

"My yoga teacher training made me able to deal and accept life's challenges; all the while learning how to share all that I learned with my students."
–Martha Watson, Devalila Yoga Teacher

Warrior Two—Option 2 Hip Opening

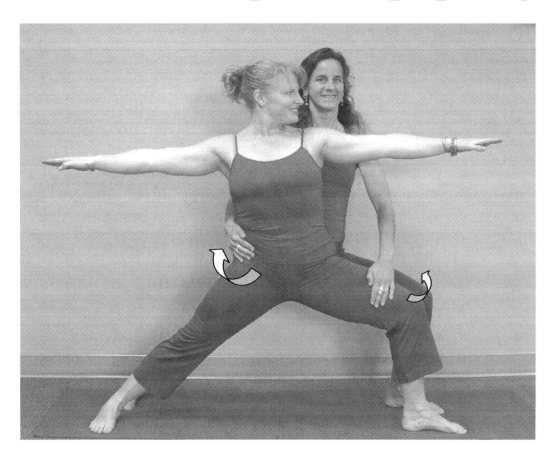

Assisting Steps for Warrior Two Pose
(Hip Opening)

Stand behind the person—practically in the same warrior stance.

Place your hand on their inner knee of the bent front leg.

Simultaneously place your other hand on the frontal pelvic crest of the hip of the back leg.

Draw the knee and hip backward toward you, but do not take the knee out of a vertical alignment with the ankle.

Maintain the assistance for as long as you feel is appropriate. Stay aware of their body and yours, and listen for their breath.

Release your hands, and allow them to return to a mountain position.

Perform the assist on the other side.

Yoga Prop Suggestions

Have them press their back foot against a wall.

What You Might Say (to help the process)

"Drop your tail bone," "Press into all parts of your feet," "Lengthen the lower back," "Let your rib cage float above the hips."

"Being assisted helps with alignment and depth, and gives a good sense of body position."
—Daniel Farrell, Devalila Yoga Teacher, Scientist

Warrior Two—Option 3 Knee Alignment

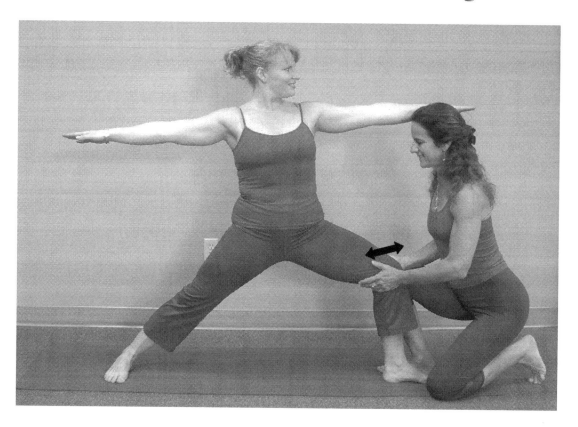

"Assisting encourages the student by making a mental note of how to get the most of the pose when they perform on their own."
–Eloise Sicora, Devalila Yoga Teacher, Pilates Teacher

Assisting Steps for Warrior Two Pose
(Knee Alignment)

Kneel in front of the person in the catcher's position.

Observe the alignment of their knee and ankle.

Use your hands to move their front knee into alignment with their ankle.

Encourage them to press firmly into both feet and keep the tail bone dropped.

Release your hands and allow them to return to a mountain position.

Perform the assist on the other side.

Yoga Prop Suggestions

Have them press their back foot against a wall.

What You Might Say (to help the process)

"Keep equal weight in both feet," "Press into all parts of your feet," "Breathe into your lower back," "Turn your hips and torso away from your front leg."

Triangle—Option 1 General Pose

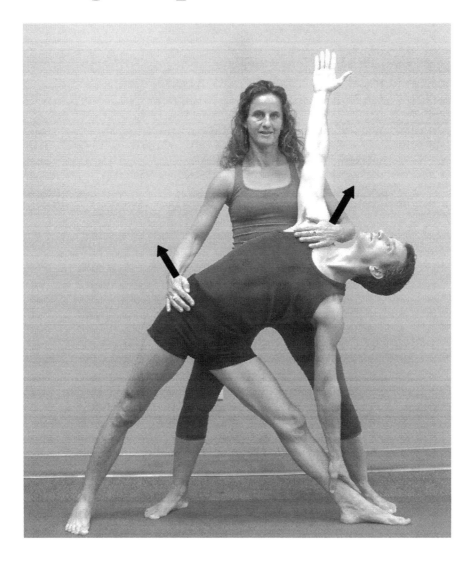

Assisting Steps for Triangle Pose (General Pose)

Stand an inch or two behind their upper back in a wide stance.

Cup their upper shoulder (front deltoid) and upper hipbone (front iliac crest) and draw them toward you.

Let your body support them as they lean slightly back into you.

Stabilize the pose by using your whole hand and a firm stance.

Deepen the assist on their exhalation.

Maintain the assistance for as long as you feel is appropriate. Stay aware of their body and yours, and listen for their breath.

Let them find their balance before you back slowly away.

Remove your hand from their hip last. Allow them to stay in the pose, or return to an upright position.

Perform the assist on the other side.

Yoga Prop Suggestions

Put a yoga block under their lower hand for support (placed near the outside of their front knee, or where ever they can reach it).

What You Might Say (to help the process)

"Position your body as if next to a wall," "Relax your shoulders," "Firmly anchor your feet," "Keep your knee and big toe in alignment," "Firm your thighs."

Triangle—Option 2 Push Pull

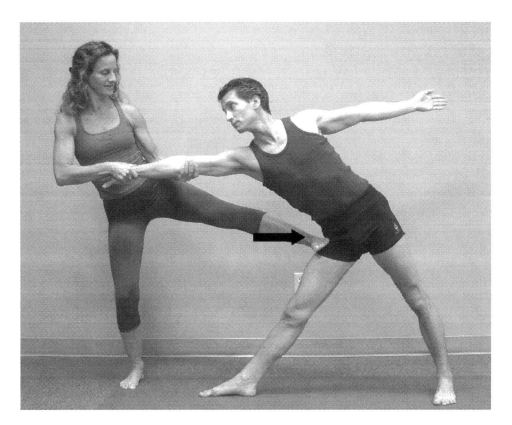

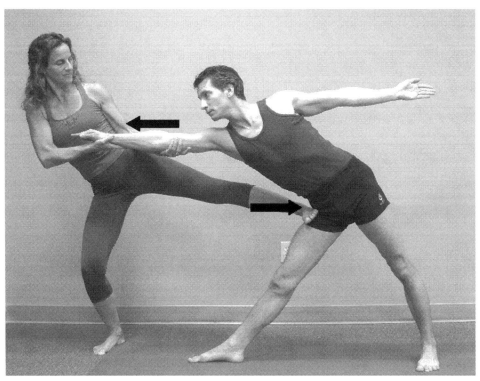

Assisting Steps for Triangle Pose (Push Pull)

Stand behind their out-stretched front hand.

Lift your leg (the one closest to them) and place the outer edge of your foot into the crease of their upper thigh.

Hold their wrist area and the area above their elbow and gently pull their arm toward you.

Simultaneously press your foot into their thigh crease (your knee will extend).

Deepen the assist on their exhalation.

Stretch them in this position until they have reached out over their front foot as much as they can.

While keeping your balance, release your foot and guide their hand downward toward their front leg (or yoga block) in the full pose.

You can now perform another triangle assist while they are in the pose.

Perform the assist on the other side.

Yoga Prop Suggestions

Put a yoga block under their lower hand for support (placed near the outside of their front knee or where they can reach it).

Have them practice the pose with the back of their body next to a wall.

What You Might Say (to help the process)

"Reach your hand forward over your front foot," "Engage your thigh muscles," "Tuck under the tail bone," "Let the weight of your hips shift backward."

Triangle—Option 3 Turning the Neck

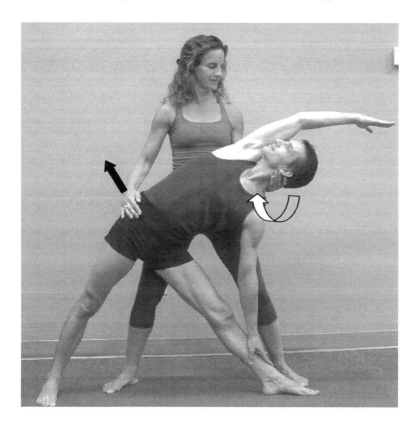

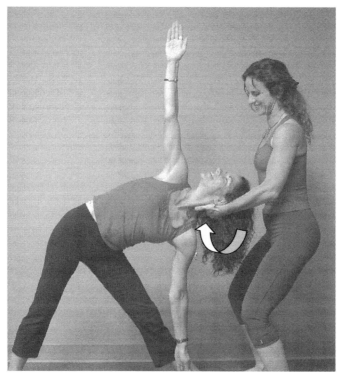

Assisting Steps for Triangle Pose
(Turning the Neck)

While assisting in the general pose, cup their neck with your whole hand for support and gently turn their head to face up (as in the top photo), or stand in front of the crown of their head in a grounded stance (as in the bottom photo).

Cradle their neck/head with both your hands around the bottom ridge of the skull (occipital ridge).

Ask them to let their head get heavy in your hands.

Guide their neck/head into alignment with the rest of their spine if it is not already.

Gently turn their head to face up and at the same time use a little traction, drawing their neck towards your body.

Maintain the assistance for as long as you feel is appropriate. Stay aware of their body and yours, and listen for their breath.

Make sure their eyes are open and they are balanced before you release your hands and move away from them.

Perform the assist on the other side.

Yoga Prop Suggestions

Put a yoga block under their lower hand for support (placed near the outside of their front knee or where they can reach it).

What You Might Say (to help the process)

"Relax your head backward in line with your spine," "Let your head get heavy."

Standing Forward Bend—Option 1
Back Pressure

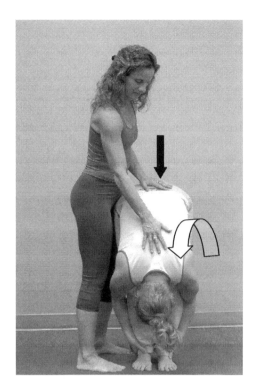

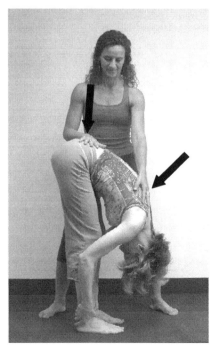

Assisting Steps for Standing Forward Bend Pose (Back Pressure)

Stand alongside the person.

Place your open hand on their sacrum for stability.

Simultaneously place your other hand in the middle of their back between the lower edges of their scapula blades.

The hand on their sacrum just stabilizes their body while the other hand presses their back down into the forward bend.

Allow them to slightly bend their knees if their belly is far from their thighs.

Maintain the assistance for as long as you feel is appropriate. Stay aware of their body and yours, and listen for their breath.

Release your hands, and allow them to return to mountain position.

Yoga Prop Suggestions

Have them press their buttocks against a wall as they fold forward.

Have them squeeze a block between their inner thighs for alignment.

What You Might Say (to help the process)

"Bend your knees," "Lean your weight forward," "Let your torso and head hang loose."

"Just when you think you have gotten your deepest in a pose, you are astonished to find that with assistance you can go even deeper." –Jessica Bayer, Devalila Yoga Teacher

Standing Forward Bend—Option 2
Body Sandwich

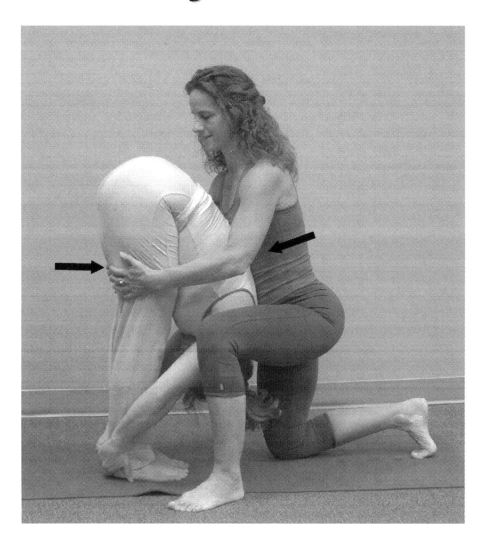

"Be authentic in your own yoga way—from your heart."
–Carrie Colditz, Devalila Yoga Teacher

Assisting Steps for Standing Forward Bend Pose (Body Sandwich)

Kneel in the marriage proposal position in front of the person's back.

Place your hands around their mid to upper hamstrings.

Simultaneously press your rib cage and belly onto their mid back.

Apply pressure between your hands and front body, sandwiching them in the forward fold.

Allow them to slightly bend their knees if their belly is far from their thighs.

Maintain the assistance for as long as you feel is appropriate. Stay aware of their body and yours, and listen for their breath.

Release your hands, stand up, and back away as they return to a mountain position.

Yoga Prop Suggestions

Have them press their buttocks against a wall as they fold forward.

Have them squeeze a block between their inner thighs for leg alignment.

What You Might Say (to help the process)

"Bend your knees," "Lean your weight into the balls of your feet," "Extend your exhale and bring your navel toward the spine," "Let your torso and head hang loosely."

Dancer

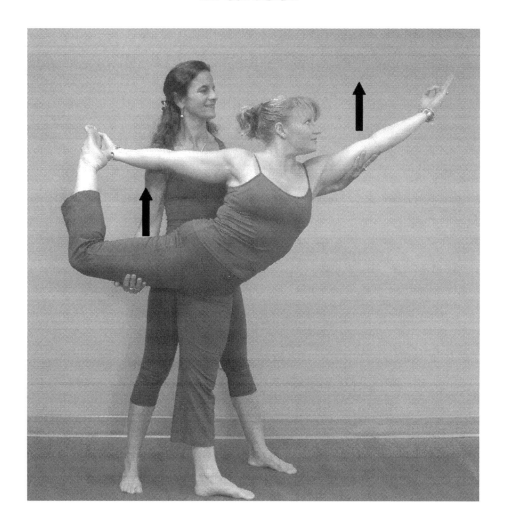

"Yoga is a dance of opposites: suppleness and strength, relaxation and vigor, lifting and grounding, darkness and light, humor and seriousness, freedom and discipline."
-Stephanie Pappas, Devalila Yoga Teacher and Trainer

Assisting Steps for Dancer Pose

Stand to the side of the person with your body lightly touching their standing leg.

One of your hands is supporting the thigh of the leg that is in the air.

Simultaneously your other hand is supporting the triceps of the arm that is in the air.

Lift their arm and leg with your hands with equal leverage.

Make sure their hips are square and their bent knee does not flare out to the side.

Maintain the assistance for as long as you feel is appropriate. Stay aware of their body and yours, and listen for their breath.

Slowly release your hands and allow them to balance on their own.

Perform the assist on the other side.

Yoga Prop Suggestions

Have them face a wall and touch it for balance.

Have them wrap a yoga tie around their ankle/foot if they cannot reach it with their hand.

What You Might Say (to help the process)

"Press your leg in the air away from your body," "Lift and expand your chest."

"Assisting leads students to self empowerment and shows them new possibilities in their bodies." –Carrie Colditz, Devalila Yoga Teacher

Half Moon One—Option 1 Sideways Stretch

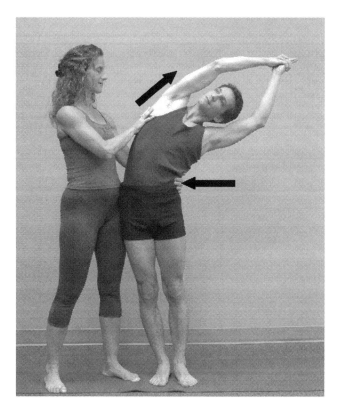

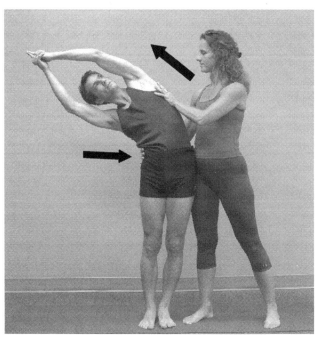

Assisting Steps for Half Moon One Pose (Sideways Stretch)

Stand on the side opposite from where they are bending with your body touching their outer hip.

Reach one of your hands around their waist and draw it toward you.

With your other hand, simultaneously press their upper rib cage in the direction they are stretching.

Apply deeper pressure on the exhalation.

Allow them to rest their head on the lower arm if they feel strain in the neck.

Maintain the assistance for as long as you feel is appropriate. Stay aware of their body and yours, and listen for their breath.

Release your hands and back away as they return mountain position.

Perform the assist on the other side.

Yoga Prop Suggestions

Have them hold a block between their hands to engage the arms.

Have them hold a yoga block between their thighs to engage the legs.

What You Might Say (to help the process)

"Reach your arms and extend the elbows," "Keep your head in alignment with your arms," "Elongate your waist area," "Breathe toward where you feel the most sensation."

Half Moon One—Option 2 Arm Pull

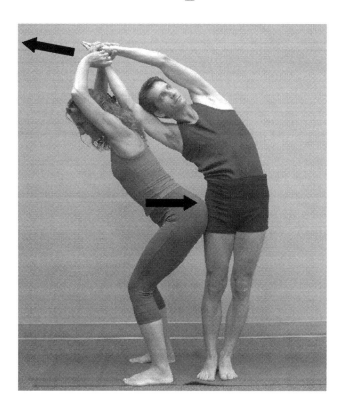

> "I feel that assisting and being assisted in the postures really helps us realize where we can go in the postures and how great it feels to be at our fullest expression of the pose. Now that I have learned what to do, it is an invaluable skill that I will use when I am teaching."
> —Jennifer Dedrick, Devalila Yoga Teacher

Assisting Steps for Half Moon One Pose (Arm Pull)

Stand in a standing squat position under their outstretched arms.

Press your buttocks into their side hip area (if you and the student have a great difference in height, this assist may not be possible).

Reach above your head and pull their wrists forward with both of your hands.

Simultaneously, push your buttocks backward against their hip and pull their arms forward.

Apply more traction on their exhalation.

Allow them to rest their head on the lower arm if they feel strain in the neck.

Maintain the assistance for as long as you feel is appropriate. Stay aware of their body and yours, and listen for their breath.

Release your hands and move away as they return to mountain position.

Perform the assist on the other side.

Yoga Prop Suggestions

Have them squeeze a block between their upper inner thighs to engage the legs.

What You Might Say (to help the process)

"Reach your arms and extend your elbows," "Keep your head in alignment with your arms," "Elongate your waist area," "Activate your leg muscles."

Half Moon Two

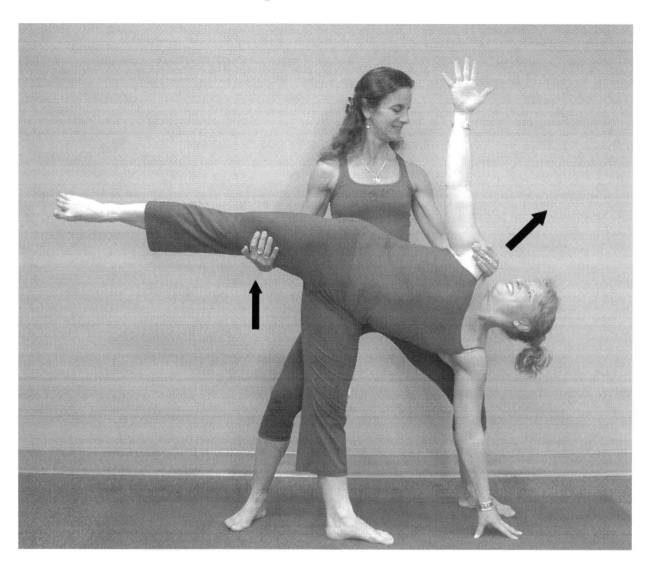

"I love assistance. It has taught me to recognize each part of my body—those parts behind
me that I cannot see, and that sometimes need to be put in place!"
–Dawn Sharp, Devalila Yoga Teacher, Personal Trainer

Assisting Steps for Half Moon Two Pose

Allow the student to get into the pose on their own as best they can.

Stand behind them with your belly or ribs (depends on their height) lightly touching their upper back around the scapula blades. Make sure your stance is wide and very stable.

Use one hand (the one nearest their leg) under the thigh that is in the air for support.

Cup your other hand (the one nearest their upper body) around the front deltoid of the arm that is in the air.

Simultaneously draw their shoulder toward your body and lift their leg toward a horizontal position in the air.

Let them lean their weight slightly backward against as if they were leaning against a wall.

Maintain the assistance for as long as you feel is appropriate. Stay aware of their body and yours, and listen for their breath.

Slowly release your hands, but remain standing there until they can balance on their own, and then back away.

Perform the assist on the other side.

Yoga Prop Suggestions

Have them place their lower hand on a yoga block.

Have them practice this pose against a wall.

What You Might Say (to help the process)

"Extend out from your navel area like a star fish," "Energize your leg in the air," "Keep your chest and hips opening," "If you feel off balance, look forward or down."

High Runner's Lunge

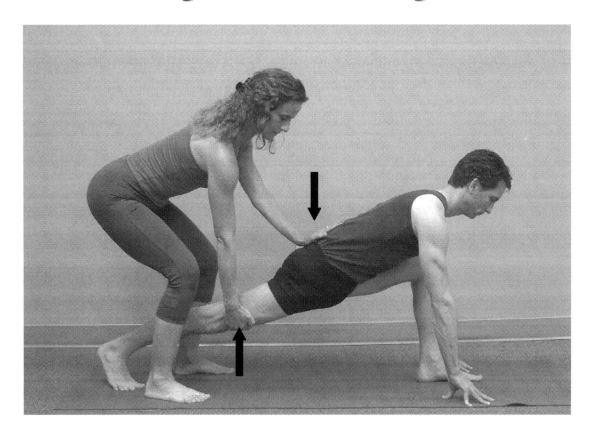

"Learning yoga was a life changing event for me. It was a gift that I hope I can continue to share with others so they may find their own sense of peace and balance."
–Michele Rodriguez, Devalila Yoga Teacher

Assisting Steps for High Runner's Lunge Pose

Straddle their back leg and bend your knees until you can reach their body.

Place one hand under their thigh above the knee area and lift upwards.

Simultaneously press down with your other hand on the middle of their sacrum.

Continue pressing down on the sacrum and lifting up on the back thigh.

Maintain the assistance for as long as you feel is appropriate. Stay aware of their body and yours, and listen for their breath.

Release your hands and allow them to bring their back leg forward and return to mountain position.

Perform the assist on the other side.

Yoga Prop Suggestions

Have them place each of their hands on yoga blocks alongside their front foot.

What You Might Say (to help the process)

"Let your hips melt toward the floor," "Extend through your back heel," "Your front knee is positioned over your ankle," "Keep your spine and neck lengthening."

"When the student feels the difference in the pose from a careful assist, the usual result is a big smile—either internal or external."—John Feist, Devalila Yoga Teacher

Pyramid

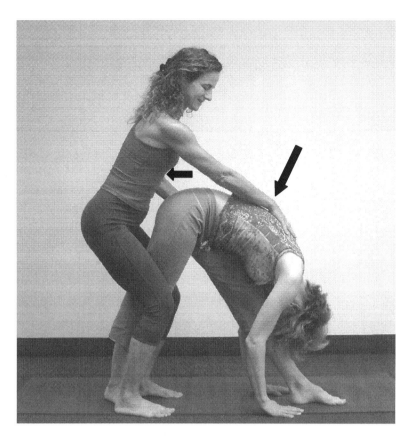

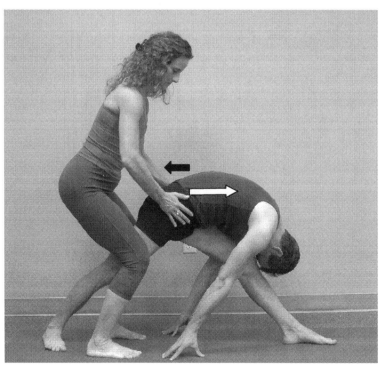

Assisting Steps for Pyramid Pose

Straddle their back leg and bend your knees in the skier's squeeze position. Firmly squeeze and stabilize their back leg with your legs.

Place one hand on their back in between the shoulder blades and press down on their exhalation.

Simultaneously with your other hand draw their hip (of the forward leg) backward. This action brings the pelvis into a more squared position.

Maintain the assistance for as long as you feel is appropriate. Stay aware of their body and yours, and listen for their breath.

Release your hands and back away as they return to mountain position.

Perform the assist on the other side.

Yoga Prop Suggestions

Have them place each of their hands on yoga blocks alongside their front leg.

What You Might Say (to help the process)

"Press firmly into both feet," "Bend your knee a bit if there is too much sensation," "Square your hips," "Let your torso relax over the front leg."

> "Stefani taught me that the fun of yoga practice often comes when you fall and laugh."
> —Ruby Hope, Yoga Teacher

Standing Yoga Mudra— Option 1
Shoulder Squeeze

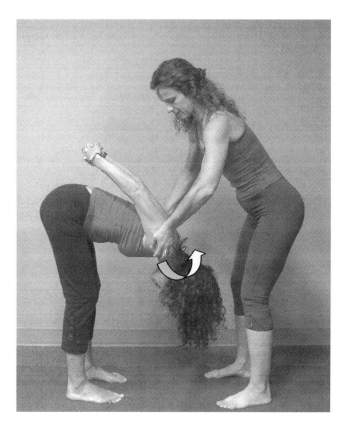

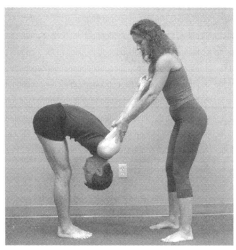

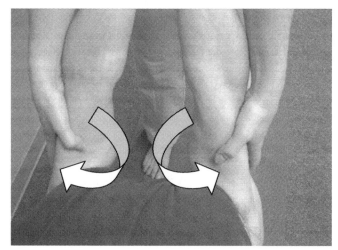

Assisting Steps for Standing Yoga Mudra Pose (Shoulder Squeeze)

Stand in front of the person's back as they are in the pose.

Begin by rolling their front shoulders inward toward their spine (as in the top photo).

Then, reach over their outstretched arms and wrap your hands around their upper arms. Your thumbs are on the inside of the arms pointing downward (as in the bottom photos).

As they exhale, firmly roll their arms toward the outside. This action should draw their shoulder blades closer together.

Continue turning their arms outward (as if you were wringing two towels) as you simultaneously draw their arms toward you (as in the bottom left photo).

Allow them to slightly bend their knees if you see that they are rounding their lower back a lot, or their belly is very far from their thighs.

Maintain the assistance for as long as you feel is appropriate. Stay aware of their body and yours, and listen for their breath.

Release your hands and allow them to return to mountain position.

Yoga Prop Suggestions

Have them hold a yoga strap between their hands if they have difficulty interlacing their fingers.

If balance is an issue, have them sit in a chair instead of standing up.

What You Might Say (to help the process)

"Bend your knees," "Squeeze your shoulder blades together," "Let your torso and head hang loose."

Standing Yoga Mudra— Option 2
Arm Stretch

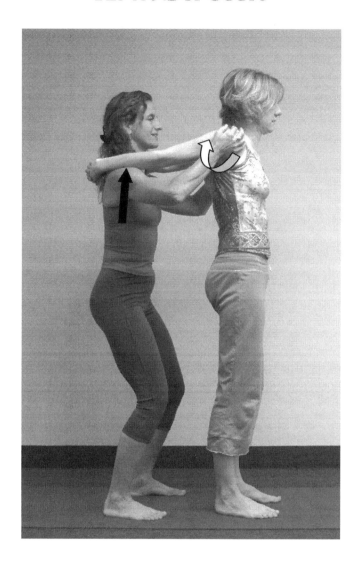

Assisting Steps for Standing Yoga Mudra Pose (Arm Stretch)

Stand in back of the person while they are in the pose with their fingers interlaced.

Bend your knees and step underneath their arms and place their forearms on your shoulders (if this is not possible, attempt another assisting variation on this pose).

As you slowly begin to stand up straighter, their arms and chest get a deep stretch.

With your hands are cupping their shoulders (deltoid area), roll them inward toward their spine. This action should bring their shoulder blades closer together.

Maintain the assistance for as long as you feel is appropriate. Stay aware of their body and yours, and listen for their breath.

Deeply bend your knees, take their arms off your shoulders and back away as they return to mountain pose.

Yoga Prop Suggestions

Have them hold a yoga strap between their hands if they have difficulty interlacing their fingers.

What You Might Say (to help the process)

"Breathe deeply into your chest," "Squeeze your shoulder blades together," "Bring your front ribs inward."

> "Cultivate an awareness of your students."
> –Carrie Colditz, Devalila Yoga Teacher

Extended Angle—Option 1 General Pose

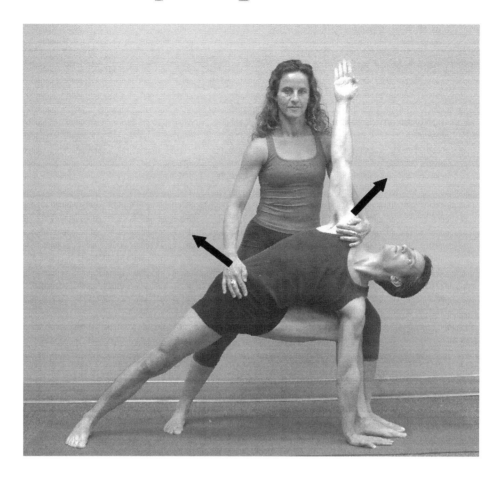

"We don't touch each other much in our society. When my students tell me how much they love the assistance I give them, it is a great reminder that physical beings like to be touched."
—Dawn Sharp, Devalila Yoga Teacher, Personal Trainer

Assisting Steps for Extended Angle Pose
(General Pose)

Stand an inch or two away from the person in a wide stance behind their middle/upper back.

Cup their upper shoulder (front deltoid) and upper hipbone (front iliac crest) with your hands and draw their body toward you.

Use your body to support them if they lean backwards into you.

Deepen the assist on their exhalation.

Maintain the assistance for as long as you feel is appropriate. Stay aware of their body and yours, and listen for their breath.

Let them find their balance before you back away.

Remove your hand from their shoulder first, then their hip, and allow them to return to an upright position.

Perform the assist on the other side.

Yoga Prop Suggestions

Have them put their lower hand on a yoga block for support (placed near the inside or outside of their front shin).

What You Might Say (to help the process)

"Position your body as if next to a wall," "Relax your shoulders,"
"Firmly anchor your feet," "Firm the buttocks muscles and tuck your tail bone,"
"Keep your knee and ankle in alignment pointing forward," "Firm your thighs."

Extended Angle—Option 2 Torso Twist

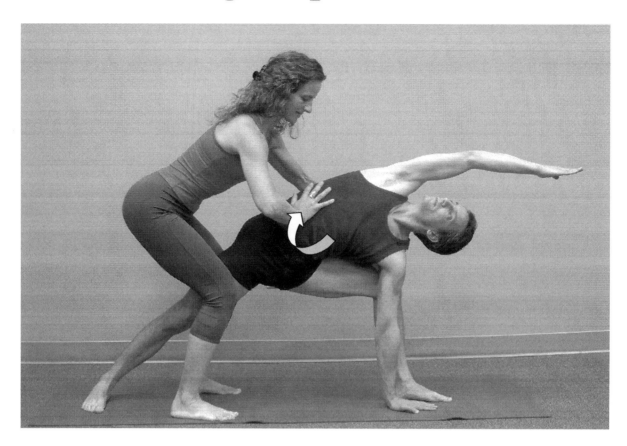

"If the assistant is stable and confident, the student may feel more secure and allow themselves to relax into the pose."
–Stephanie Pappas, Devalila Yoga Teacher and Trainer

Assisting Steps for Extended Angle Pose
(Torso Twist)

Straddle their back leg and bend your knees in the skier's squeeze position. Firmly squeeze and stabilize their back leg with your legs.

Place one hand on the lower part of their scapula blade (the one that is closest to the floor). This hand will press the scapula in a downward direction.

Simultaneously place your other hand (fingers facing away from their navel) on their rib cage (the ribs that are facing the sky).

Twist their torso with both your hands, moving in a direction away from their navel.

Twist more deeply on their exhalation and intensify your grip on their back leg.

Maintain the assistance for as long as you feel is appropriate. Stay aware of their body and yours, and listen for their breath.

Release your hands and let them twist on their own. Slowly back away as they return to an upright position.

Perform the assist on the other side.

Yoga Prop Suggestions

Have them put their lower hand on a yoga block for support (placed near the inside or outside of their front shin).

What You Might Say (to help the process)

"Press firmly into both feet," "Tuck the tail bone under and firm the buttocks," "Open your chest and armpit toward the ceiling," "Press your bottom arm backward against your knee for leverage in the twist."

Warrior Three

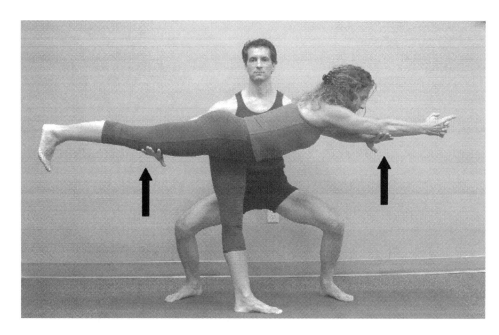

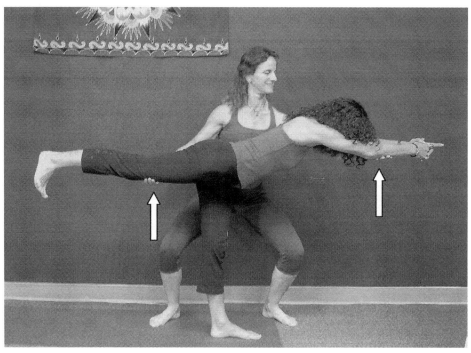

Assisting Steps for Warrior Three Pose

Stand alongside the person in a horse stance near their standing leg (slightly in contact with their body).

Use one of your hands (back of your hand or palm) to support and lift the thigh of the leg that is in the air.

Simultaneously use your other hand (back of your hand or palm) to support and lift the arms that are in the air.

Without moving them off balance, lift their arms and leg with your hands so that their body is approaching a "T" position.

Maintain the assistance for as long as you feel is appropriate. Stay aware of their body and yours, and listen for their breath.

Slowly release your hands and back away.

Allow them to balance on their own before they return to mountain position.

Perform the assist on the other side.

Yoga Prop Suggestions

Allow them to face a wall or a chair and touch it for balance.

Have them press their back foot into a wall.

What You Might Say (to help the process)

"Extend your leg in the air," "Firm the standing leg," "Align your leg, arms, and your torso," "Bring your navel toward your spine as you exhale."

> "A student may remember a feather suggestion for weeks."
> —Carrie Colditz, Devalila Yoga Teacher

Standing Split—Option 1 Leg Lift

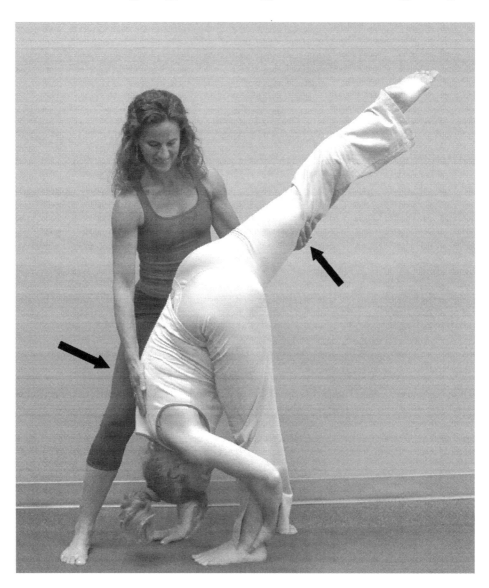

Assisting Steps for Standing Leg Split Pose
(Leg Lift)

Stand alongside the person in a wide stance (on the side with the leg in the air).

Place one hand on the middle of their front thigh of the leg in the air. Place the other hand on the middle of their back between the shoulder blades.

Simultaneously press down on the middle of their back as you lift their standing leg higher.

Allow them to slightly bend the knee of the standing leg if you see that their belly is very far from their thighs.

Maintain the assistance for as long as you feel is appropriate. Stay aware of their body and yours, and listen for their breath.

Release your hands and back away as they bring their legs together and return to mountain position.

Perform the assist on the other side.

Yoga Prop Suggestions

Have them place their lower hand(s) on a block(s) for support.

What You Might Say (to help the process)

"Reach your legs in equal and opposite directions," "Point your toes toward the ceiling," "Relax your neck."

"What force in the lightest of touches."
—Carrie Colditz, Devalila Yoga Teacher

Standing Split—Option 2 Body Sandwich

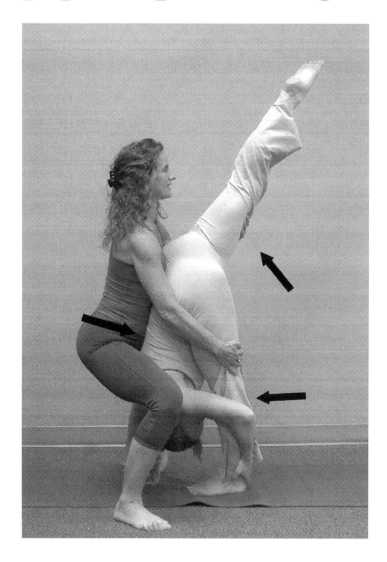

"Yoga showed me the door to ultimate happiness and peace of body and mind."
-Varsha Patel, Devalila Yoga Teacher

Assisting Steps for Standing Leg Split Pose (Body Sandwich)

Stand in a deep squat position in front of the person's back.

Place one hand on the middle to upper hamstrings of their lower leg.

Place the other hand under the knee or thigh of their upper leg and apply a lift.

Simultaneously press your rib cage and belly onto the middle of their back as you pull their standing leg toward you.

Apply pressure between your hands and front body, sandwiching them in the standing split.

Allow them to slightly bend their knee if you see that their belly is very far from their thighs.

Maintain the assistance for as long as you feel is appropriate. Stay aware of their body and yours, and listen for their breath.

Release your hands, stand up, and back away as they bring their legs together and return to mountain position.

Perform the assist on the other side.

Yoga Prop Suggestions

Have them place their lower hand(s) on a block(s) for support.

What You Might Say (to help the process)

"Reach your legs in equal and opposite directions," "Point your toes toward the ceiling."

Seated Forward Folding Hip and Leg Postures

Seated posture adjustments are somewhat easier to perform because there is no risk of knocking the person over as there is in the standing postures, and you are working with gravity. Because the person is in a seated position, you have more time to set up and position yourself. The challenge of adjusting a seated forward fold pose is to know how much pressure to apply. You may have some apprehension in the beginning. With time and practice you will gain confidence about the level of pressure to apply. Here are some points to remember when assisting someone in the forward folding poses presented in this chapter:

- Have the person bend their knees a little or a lot when they have tight hamstrings.

- Have props handy and ready to give them for support under the knees, belly, or buttocks.

- If you are unsure of the appropriate amount of pressure to apply, ask for specific feedback.

- Don't force the student into the fold. If you feel resistance and they are not breathing, back off.

- Apply pressure gradually and in harmony with their breath.

- Apply deeper pressure on their exhalation.

- When pressing on their back or spine, use your whole hand.

- When pressing on their back or spine with both your hands, use equal pressure in both hands.

Note: All the postures in the following section should be performed for at least 30 seconds, but can be held for much longer depending on the needs and ability of the student.

Seated Forward Fold—Props

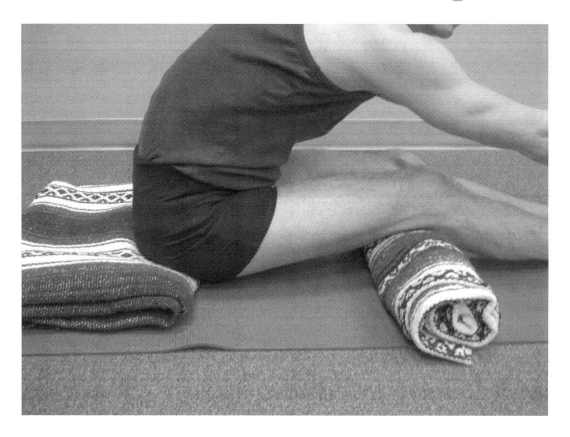

"Just relax and let the pose find its expression in you..." –Joy Principe, C.P.A., Yoga Teacher

Yoga Prop suggestions for Seated Forward Folding Poses

You can place a folded blanket or a pillow under your hips.

Remember to sit on the <u>edge</u> of the blanket or pillow and not directly in the middle of it.

You can place a rolled-up blanket, a round bolster, or small to medium size pillow under the knees to relax the hamstring muscles.

You can press your feet against a wall to give your legs an extra stretch.

If no props are available for under your hips you can roll up your yoga mat and sit on that.

If no props are available for under your knees you can slide your forearms under you knees for support, or simply keep your knees slightly bent.

"Assisting is about reminding a person that it's ok to let go and really enjoy the pose."
–Joy Principe, C.P.A., Yoga Teacher

Seated Forward Fold—Option 1
Rib Cage Lift and Press

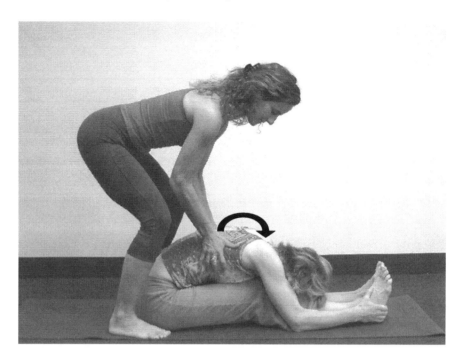

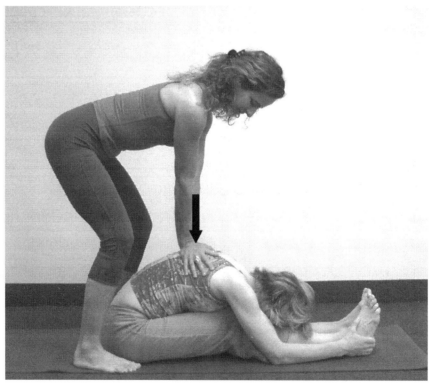

Assisting Steps for Forward Fold Pose
(Rib Cage Lift and Press)

Stand in a standing squat position close to the person's back with your feet near the outside of their hips.

Place your hands firmly around the sides of their middle/lower rib cage and trace your fingers around their ribs.

As they inhale, lift their rib cage up and slightly forward (as in the top photo).

As they exhale, press their rib cage down and slightly forward with equal pressure in both hands (as in the bottom photo).

Perform the lift and press several times, synchronizing your movements with their breath.

Maintain the assistance for as long as you feel is appropriate. Stay aware of their body and yours, and listen for their breath.

Release your hands, stand up, and back away as they roll up to a seated position.

Yoga Prop Suggestions

Have them put a pillow under their hips, belly, or knees for support.

Have them press their feet into a wall for a deeper leg stretch.

What You Might Say (to help the process)

"Relax your neck, arms and shoulders," "Reach your navel toward your thighs," "Let go and let gravity take you deeper into the fold."

Seated Forward Fold—Option 2 Sacrum Tilt

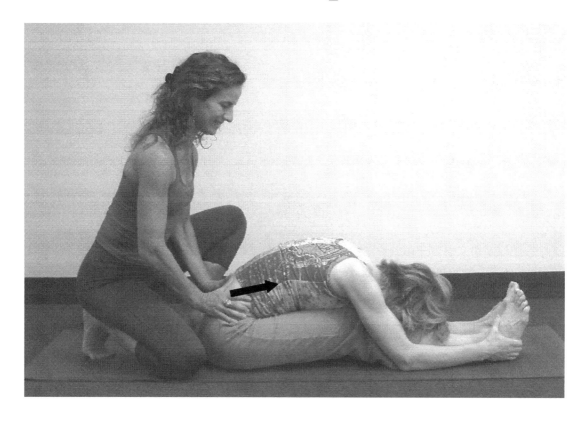

"When the teacher is assisting you, breathe deeply and melt into the pose."
-Stephanie Pappas, Devalila Yoga Teacher and Trainer

Assisting Steps for Forward Fold Pose (Sacrum Tilt)

Kneel in the catcher's position close to the person's back.

Place the heels of your hands firmly on their lower back/sacrum area with your fingers facing upward and slightly outward (it depends on what feels comfortable to you).

Maintain a continuous, even pressure downward and slightly forward on their sacrum.

As they breathe and relax in the pose, you can shift the position of your hands an inch or two (up, down or laterally) and continue applying pressure.

Maintain the assistance for as long as you feel is appropriate. Stay aware of their body and yours, and listen for their breath.

Release your hands, stand up, and back away as they roll up to a seated position.

Yoga Prop Suggestions

Have them put a pillow under their hips, belly, or knees for support.

Have them press their feet into a wall for a deeper leg stretch.

What You Might Say (to help the process)

"Tilt your pelvis forward," "Press your hips toward the floor," "Reach your navel toward your thighs," "Keep your feet and legs together."

"Help your students find joy in their practice."
—Carrie Colditz, Devalila Yoga Teacher

85

Seated Forward Fold—Option 3
Light Pressure

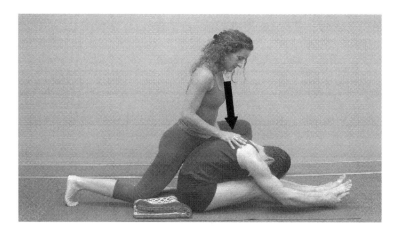

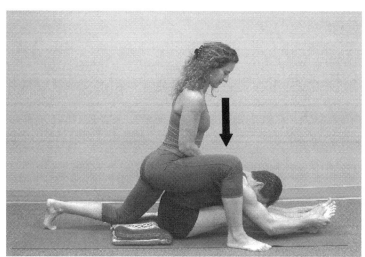

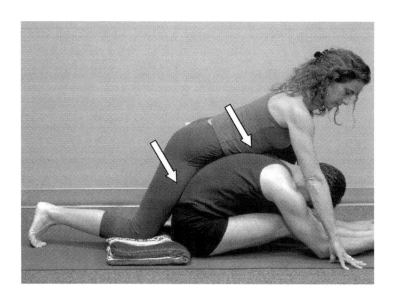

Assisting Steps for Forward Fold Pose
(Light Pressure)

Kneel close to the person's back and place one of your feet near the outside of their thigh or knee (whichever feels more comfortable to you). Let your other leg extend backward into a low lunge position.

Place your hands firmly on their middle back in the area between or beneath the scapula blades.

As they inhale, ease up on the pressure.

As they exhale, press down and slightly forward with equal pressure in both hands.

If they can (or want to) go deeper, shift your weight forward and lean your rib cage, belly, and upper thigh onto their back (as in the bottom photo). Apply pressure with your whole body as they exhale.

Put your hands on the floor for balance.

Maintain the assist for as long as you feel is appropriate.

Return to an upright position and back away as they roll up to a seated position.

Yoga Prop Suggestions

Have them put a pillow under their hips, belly, or knees for support.

What You Might Say (to help the process)

"Relax your neck, arms, and shoulders," "Relax more as you exhale," Keep your feet flexed."

Seated Forward Fold—Option 4
Deep Pressure Using Torso and Hand

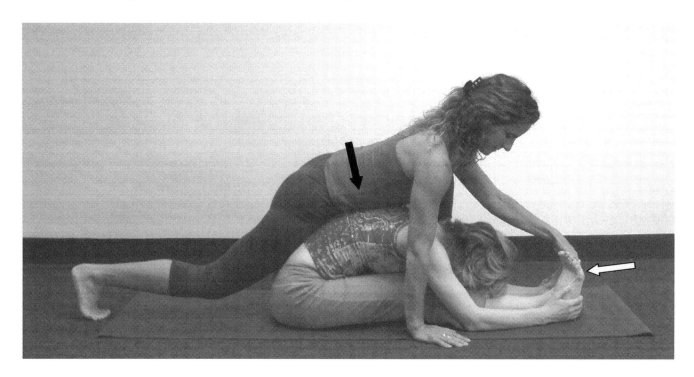

"After receiving assistance with the forward fold it was amazing to me how much deeper I could go in the pose on my own! It was as if I continued to feel hands lifting up my abdomen each time I took a breath, and on the releasing sinking me down."
–Michele Lawrence, Devalila Yoga Teacher

Assisting Steps for Forward Fold Pose (Deep Pressure Using Torso and Hand)

NOTE: Use this assist if the person still wants to go deeper after receiving the previous forward fold assists.

Place one of your feet near the outside of their thigh or knee. Let your other leg extend backward into a low lunge position.

Shift your weight onto your front foot and then lean your upper thigh, your belly, and lastly your ribs onto their back.

Simultaneously place your hand (or hands) on the floor alongside their legs for balance.

Apply more pressure on their exhale by lifting your back knee off the floor and leaning your weight forward and down onto their back.

When you feel balanced, use one of your hands to flex their feet forward.

Maintain the assistance for as long as you feel is appropriate. Stay aware of their body and yours, and listen for their breath.

Remove your hands, return to a kneeling position, and back away as they roll up to a seated position.

Yoga Prop Suggestions

Have them put a pillow under their hips or knees for support.

If they are really flexible have them hold onto a yoga block at the bottoms of their feet.

What You Might Say (to help the process)

"Relax completely, but keep your feet flexed," "Let go more as you exhale."

Seated Forward Fold—Option 5
Back-to-Back

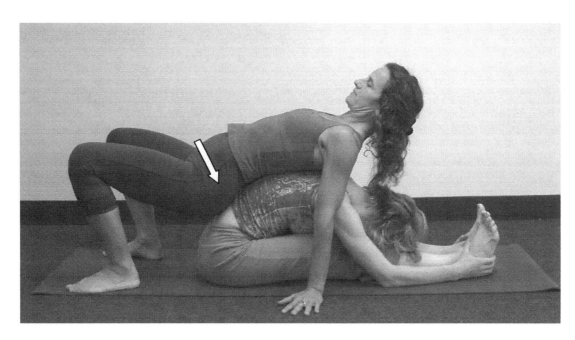

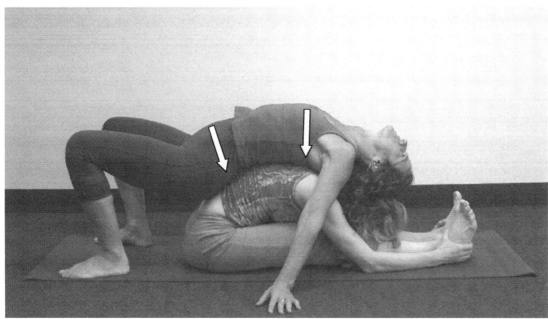

Assisting Steps for Forward Fold Pose
(Back-to-Back)

Sit down near their hips with your back facing theirs and your knees bent. Place your feet on the floor about hip width apart.

Place your hands flat on the floor behind you.

Lift your hips off the floor and place your low back/sacrum area onto their low back/sacrum area.

Slowly, press your back onto their back and maintain full contact and alignment.

As you lean backward over their body, adjust your hand position to maintain your balance and stability.

Maintain the assistance for as long as you feel is appropriate. Stay aware of their body and yours, and listen for their breath.

Release by rolling your spine up starting with your head and ending with your low back. Slide your hips back down to the floor into a seated position as they roll up from the forward fold.

Yoga Prop Suggestions

Place a blanket between your back and their back to soften the bone to bone contact.

What You Might Say (to help the process)

"Do you want more or less pressure?" "Relax and deepen your breath as I lean my weight onto you."

Child—Option 1 Sacrum Press

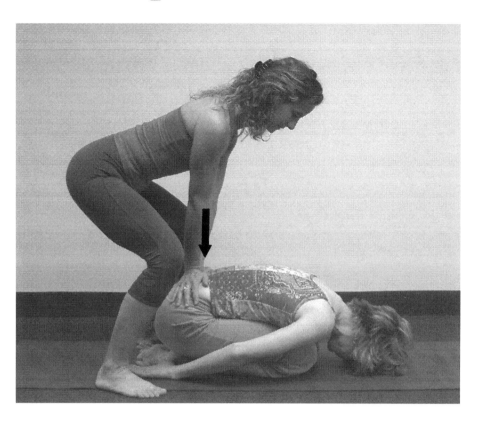

"My yoga teacher's assistance resembles a parent helping a child getting on their feet in early years of life."
-Varsha Patel, Devalila Yoga Teacher

Assisting Steps for Child's Pose (Sacrum Press)

Stand with bent knees close to the person's back and your feet hip width apart.

Place your hands firmly on their sacrum area with your fingers facing out to the sides. Your wrists are centered in the middle of their sacrum.

While keeping your arms straight, bend your knees more and press down onto their sacrum using your body weight.

Maintain equal pressure on their inhalation and exhalation.

Maintain the assistance for as long as you feel is appropriate. Stay aware of their body and yours, and listen for their breath.

Release your hands, stand up, and back away as they roll up to a seated position.

Yoga Prop Suggestions

Have them spread their knees apart or put a pillow under their belly for support.

Have them put a pillow or blanket between their hips and their feet.

What You Might Say (to help the process)

"Breathe deeply into your diaphragm and lower back," "Relax your shoulders."

> "I'm looking forward to introducing yoga to my daughter. I know she will love it especially since she experienced it in the womb!"
> —Michele Rodriguez, Devalila Yoga Teacher

Child—Option 2
Sacrum Press with Arm Stretch

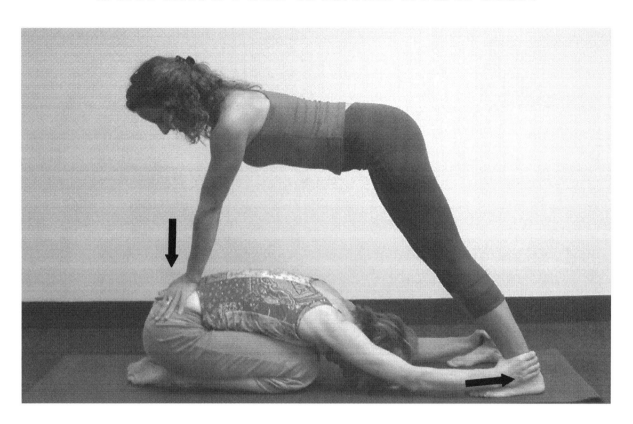

"With the teacher's assistance during class, I was able to go beyond where I was in the pose and have a 'template' of what is possible for me to stretch into with further practice. This is a metaphor for life also."
–Madonna Alvarez, Devalila Yoga Student

Assisting Steps for Child's Pose
(Sacrum Press with Arm Stretch)

Stand with bent knees close to the person's extended arms and let them hold onto your ankles with a firm grip.

Reach over their back and place your hands firmly on their sacrum area with your fingers facing out to the sides. Your wrists are centered in the middle of their sacrum.

While keeping your arms straight, press down onto their sacrum using your body weight. Really lean forward as if you were going to do a push up with your shoulders almost over your wrists.

Step your feet backwards one at a time to give their arms a deeper stretch.

Maintain the assistance for as long as you feel is appropriate. Stay aware of their body and yours, and listen for their breath.

Bend your knees, release your hands and stand up straight. Ask them to release your ankles.

Yoga Prop Suggestions

Have them spread their knees apart, or put a pillow under their belly for support.

Have them put a pillow or blanket between their hips and their feet.

What You Might Say (to help the process)

"Breathe deeply into your diaphragm and lower back," "Hold firmly onto my ankles and relax your shoulders."

Head to Knee Fold

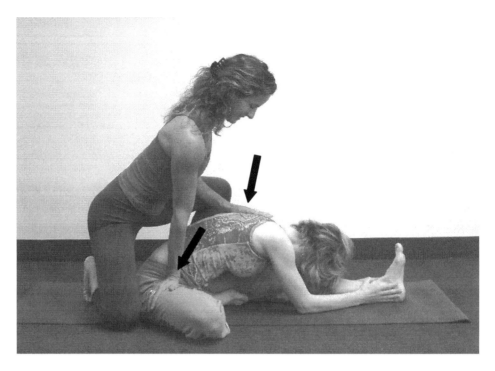

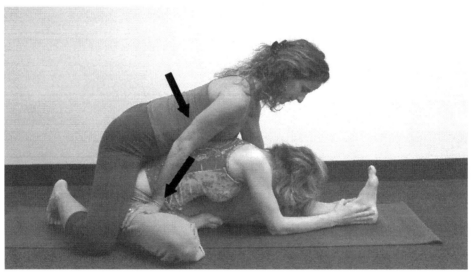

Assisting Steps for Head to Knee Fold Pose

NOTE: You can perform the rib cage lift and press before doing the following steps.

Kneel close to the person's back in the catcher's position (or a standing squat position).

Place the heel of one your hands on their bent leg close to the leg crease, and apply pressure. Your fingers are pointing away from their groin area.

Place your other hand on the center of their back between the lower scapula blades, and gradually apply pressure with each exhalation.

Simultaneously apply pressure on both areas, but lighten the pressure on their back during the inhalation.

Maintain the assistance for as long as you feel is appropriate.

Release your hands, stand up, and back away as they roll up to a seated position.

Perform the assist on the other side.

Yoga Prop Suggestions

Have them put a pillow under one or both knees for support.

Have them press their foot into a wall for a deeper leg stretch.

What You Might Say (to help the process)

"Relax your neck, arms, and shoulders," "Reach your navel toward your thighs."

Half Hero Fold

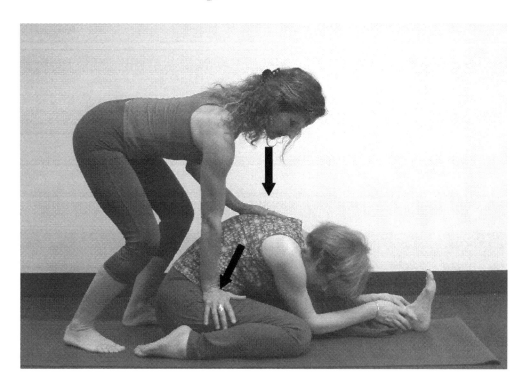

"My yoga teacher training had an incredible impact on my life. On the one hand it softened me; on the other hand it made me stronger."
–Martha Watson, Devalila Yoga Teacher

Assisting Steps Half Hero Fold Pose

NOTE: *You can perform the rib cage lift and press before doing the following steps.*

Stand in a standing squat position close to the person's back(or kneel in the catcher's position).

Place the heel of one of your hands on their bent leg close to the leg crease, and apply pressure. Your fingers are pointing away from their groin area.

Place your other hand on the center of their back between the lower scapula blades, and gradually apply pressure with each exhalation.

Simultaneously apply pressure on both areas, but lighten the pressure on their back during the inhalation.

Release your hands, stand up, and back away as they roll up to a seated position.

Perform the assist on the other side.

Yoga Prop Suggestions

Have them put a pillow under the knee of the extended leg for support.

Have them press their foot into a wall for a deeper leg stretch.

What You Might Say (to help the process)

"Relax your neck, arms and shoulders," "Reach your navel toward your thighs."

Cobbler

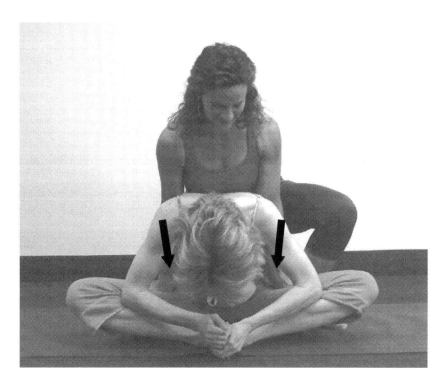

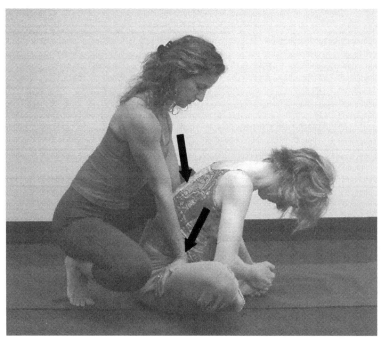

Assisting Steps for Cobbler's Pose

NOTE: You can perform the rib cage lift and press before doing the following steps.

Kneel close to the person's back in the catcher's position (or a standing squat position).

Press the heels of your hands down on their legs (close to the thigh creases) and gradually apply pressure. Your fingers should be pointing away from the groin area.

Anchor their legs down with a steady pressure as they breathe and fold forward.

Maintain the assistance for as long as you feel is appropriate.

Release your hands, stand up, and back away as they roll up to a seated position.

Yoga Prop Suggestions

Have them put pillows under both knees for support.

Have them sit on the edge of a blanket or pillow.

If they are really flexible, have them press a yoga block between their feet.

What You Might Say (to help the process)

"Fold forward from your hip crease," "Reach your navel toward the floor," "Relax your neck and shoulders," "Press your heels together."

"I really appreciate the willingness and openness of my students."
–Stephanie Pappas, Devalila Yoga Teacher and Trainer

Seated Wide Spread Fold

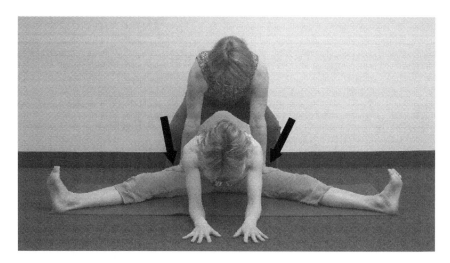

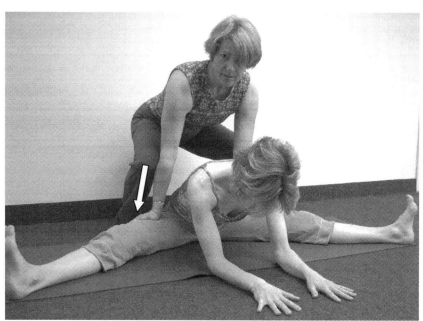

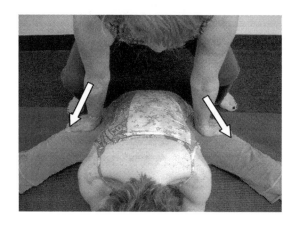

Assisting Steps for Seated Wide Spread Fold Pose

Note: You can perform the rib cage lift and press before doing the following steps.

Stand close to the person's back in the standing squat position (or kneel in the catcher's position).

Press the heels of your hands down on their legs (close to the thigh creases) and gradually apply pressure. Your fingers are pointing away from their groin area.

Anchor their legs down with a steady pressure as they breathe and fold forward.

Maintain the assistance for as long as you feel is appropriate.

Release your hands, stand up, and back away as they roll up to a seated position.

Yoga Prop Suggestions

Have them put a pillow under both knees for support.

Have them sit on the edge of a blanket or pillow.

What You Might Say (to help the process)

"Fold forward from your hip crease," "Reach your navel toward the floor," "Relax your neck and shoulders," "Flex your feet and engage your thighs."

Other Hip and Leg Postures

There are so many great leg and hip postures. In this chapter I decided to focus on some of the most common hip and leg postures (in addition to the forward folding postures shown in the previous chapter).

Here are some points to remember when assisting someone in the hip and leg poses in this chapter of the book. They are quite similar to the points in the previous chapter:

- Have the person bend their knees during a pose if they have tight hamstring muscles.

- Use yoga props to provide support and comfort to people who have tension in their lower back and hip muscles.

- Use your whole hand and not just your fingers during the posture adjustments.

- Use your body weight and gravity versus muscle strength when applying pressure.

- Find a balance between too much and too little pressure.

- Ask for specific feedback about the level of pressure they desire.

- Apply pressure gradually and in harmony with their breath.

- Deepen the pressure on their exhalation.

Note: All the postures in the following section should be performed for at least 30 seconds, but can be held for much longer depending on the needs and ability of the student.

Hero

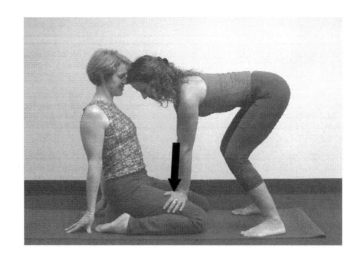

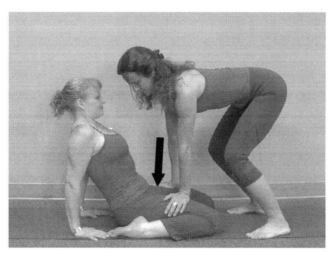

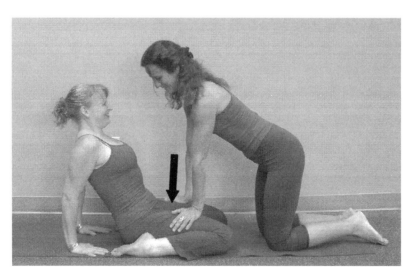

Assisting Steps for Hero Pose

Stand in front of the person's legs in a standing squat position (as in the top photos), or kneel in front of their legs (bottom photo).

Place your hands down on their thighs above the knee area.

Gradually press the heels of your hands down on their legs. Your fingers are pointing toward the outsides of the legs.

Slowly walk your hands up the thighs toward the thigh crease. Lean your weight into one hand and then the other, in a slow rocking motion.

Slowly walk your hands back down the thighs toward the knee area. Lean your weight into one hand and then the other, in a slow rocking motion.

Repeat the technique as many times as you feel is appropriate.

Release your hands, stand up, and back away as release the position of their legs.

Yoga Prop Suggestions

Have them sit on the edge of a blanket or pillow.

Have them kneel on a soft, flat blanket.

What You Might Say (to help the process)

"Align your heels with your big toes," "Spread your knees further apart if you have any knee pain," "Sit on a pillow if you feel any knee pain," "Sit up tall and keep your navel reaching toward your spine."

Heron

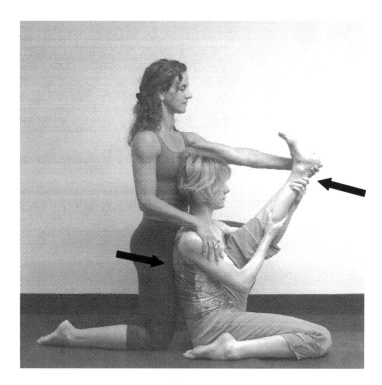

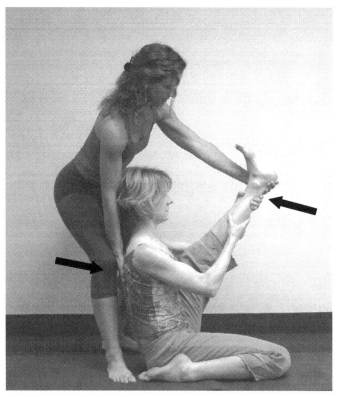

Assisting Steps for Heron Pose

Kneel close to the person's back in the marriage proposal position with the front of your thigh aligned with their spine so that you are supporting their back (as in the top photo).

You can also stand with your inner shin aligned with the spine, and use your hand to support their upper back (as in the bottom photo).

Use your other hand to hold the ankle of their outstretched leg and gradually draw it toward their torso.

Maintain the assistance for as long as you feel is appropriate.

Release your hand, stand, and back away as they release their leg to the floor.

Perform the assist on the other side.

Yoga Prop Suggestions

Have them sit on the edge of a blanket or pillow.

What You Might Say (to help the process)

"Lengthen your spine, especially your lower back" "Relax your neck and shoulders," "Draw your leg toward you without leaning backwards."

"Yoga practice increases our awareness of feelings and the whole range of human experiences. We are nailed to the present moment and there is nowhere to hide."
–Stephanie Pappas, Devalila Yoga Teacher and Trainer

Leg Cradle

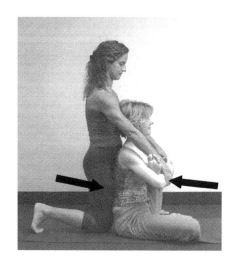

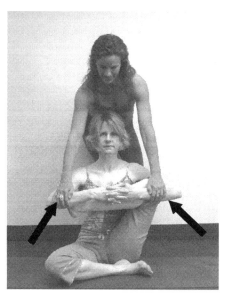

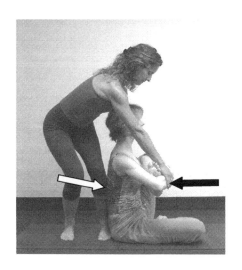

Assisting Steps for Leg Cradle Pose

Kneel close to the person's back in the marriage proposal position with the front of your thigh aligned with their spine so that you are supporting their back (as in the top photo).

You can also stand with your inner shin aligned with the spine to support their upper back (as in the bottom photos).

Use your hands to pull the shin of their bent leg toward their torso.

Maintain the assistance for as long as you feel is appropriate.

Release your hands, stand up, and back away as they release the leg position.

Perform the assist on the other side.

Yoga Prop Suggestions

Have them sit on the edge of a blanket or pillow.

What You Might Say (to help the process)

"Lengthen your spine, especially your lower back," "Bring your shin toward your chest," "Draw your leg toward you without leaning backwards."

"For me yoga is the most satisfying type of exercise imaginable."
–Amy Hentenaar, Yoga Student

Squat

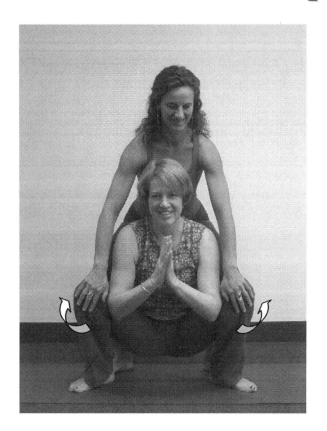 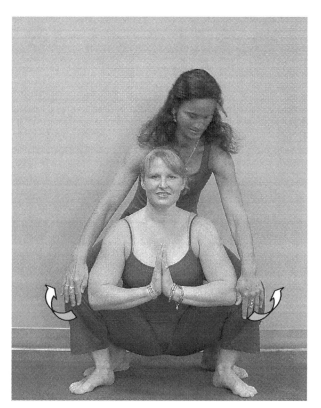

"To assist someone takes patience, centeredness and caring— without these qualities, it is just touching."
–Adrienne Yurinko, Devalila Yoga Teacher

Assisting Steps for Squat Pose

Stand close to the person's back in a standing squat position.

Use your hands to slowly draw their knees backward without moving them out of alignment with their ankles.

Maintain the assistance for as long as you feel is appropriate.

Release your hands and back away as they return to a standing position.

Yoga Prop Suggestions

Have them sit on a yoga block or two.

Place a rolled up blanket, yoga mat, or yoga wedges under their heels (if their heels don't easily touch the ground).

What You Might Say (to help the process)

"Lengthen your spine, especially your upper back," "Press your elbows into your inner knees," "Drop your shoulders and open your chest area."

"Not only does yoga offer the physical challenge of 'perfecting' or refining the various movements and postures, but with the right instructor or 'facilitator' yoga provides a far more valuable mind-body-spirit connection." –Amy Hentenaar, Yoga Student

Downward Dog—Option 1 Sacrum Press

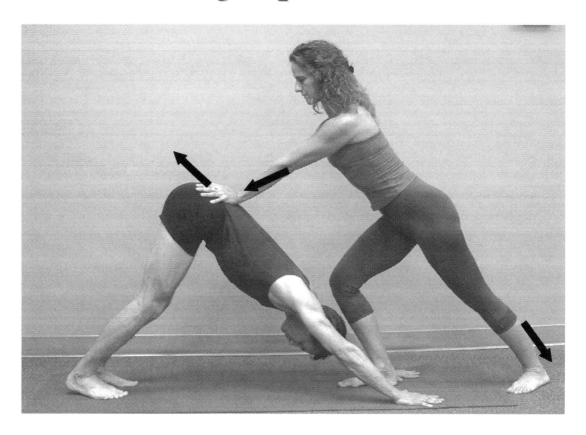

"It just feels right to have every bit of my body increasingly stretched in downward dog pose."
–Carrie Colditz, Devalila Yoga Teacher

Assisting Steps for Downward Dog Pose
(Sacrum Press)

Stand in front of the person in a lunge type position with your foot between their hands.

You can also stand in a standing squat position with your feet beside their hands.

Place the heels of your hands firmly down on their sacrum area with your fingers facing upward and slightly outward.

Press into your feet into the floor and lean your body weight forward without bending your arms.

Maintain a continuous, even pressure downward and slightly upward on their sacrum.

As they breathe and hold the pose, you can shift your hand position an inch or two (up, down, or laterally) and continue applying pressure.

Maintain the assistance for as long as you feel is appropriate.

Perform a different assist for downward dog pose, or release your hands and allow them to return to mountain position.

Yoga Prop Suggestions

Have them press their heels up on a wall.

Have them squeeze a yoga block between their thighs.

Have them place their hands on yoga blocks.

What You Might Say (to help the process)

"Breathe deeply into your upper chest and diaphragm," "Press down into your palms," "Look toward your navel," "Drop your shoulders away from your ears."

Downward Dog—Option 2 Leg Pull

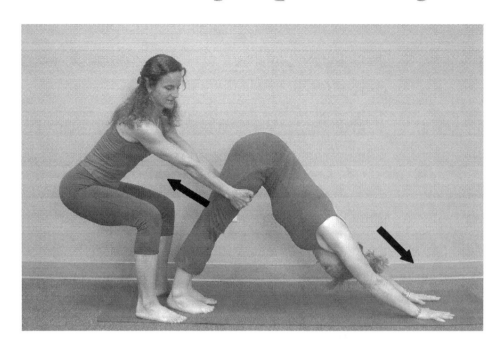

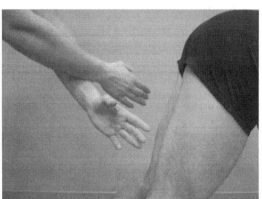

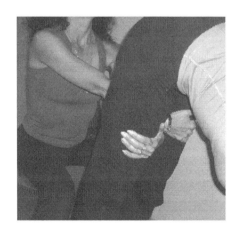

Assisting Steps for Downward Dog Pose
(Leg Pull)

Stand in a standing squat position in back of the person with your feet spread apart wider than theirs.

Wrap your hands firmly around the biggest part of their front thighs (as in the top photo), or cross one of your wrists over the other and reach through the inside of their thighs to hold onto the biggest part of their front thighs (as in the bottom photos).

Lean of all your weight backward into your hips as if you were sitting into a chair.

Keep your arms straight and allow your knees to bend more as you hold firmly onto their upper thighs.

Maintain the assistance for as long as you feel is appropriate.

Perform a different assist for downward dog pose, or release your hands and allow them to return to mountain position.

Yoga Prop Suggestions

Have them squeeze a yoga block between their thighs.

Have them place their hands on yoga blocks.

What You Might Say (to help the process)

"Reach your hips toward the sky," "Press down into your palms," "Draw your knees caps up and firm your thighs," "Reach your heels toward the floor."

Downward Dog—Option 3 Heel Press

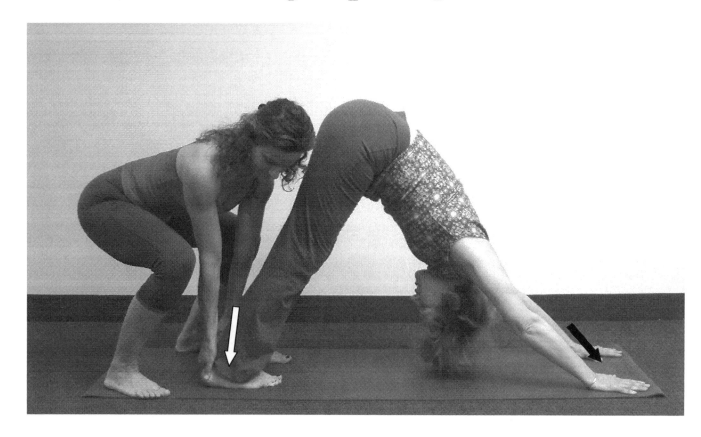

"Assisting is crucial to helping a student get the most from a pose."
—John Feist, Devalila Yoga Teacher

Assisting Steps for Downward Dog Pose
(Heel Press)

Stand in a deep squat position in back of the person with your feet spread apart wider than theirs.

Stretch their heels toward the floor by firmly squeezing them between your thumbs and index fingers (thumbs are on the outer heels) and pressing downward.

Keep your arms straight.

Sink your body weight downward toward the floor as you bend your knees more.

Maintain the assistance for as long as you feel is appropriate.

Perform a different assist for downward dog pose, or release your hands and allow them to return to mountain position.

Yoga Prop Suggestions

Have them squeeze a yoga block between their thighs.

Have them place their hands on yoga blocks.

What You Might Say (to help the process)

"Reach your hips toward the sky," "Press down into your palms," "Draw your knees caps up and firm your thighs," "Reach your heels toward the floor."

"I have found that some people don't like to be corrected in a posture even if it is for their own good. They stiffen up and resist the assist." –John Feddersen, Devalila Yoga Teacher

Pigeon Preparation—Option 1 Sacrum Press

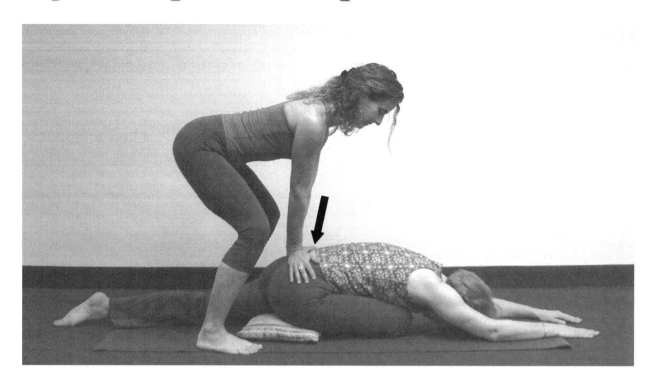

"A class is not supposed to be the same as a personal practice. Class is time for students to learn new poses and find ways to get deeper into poses than they may already be practicing."
—John Feist, Devalila Yoga Teacher

Assisting Steps for Pigeon Preparation Pose (Sacrum Press)

Straddle their back leg in a standing squat position with your feet about hip width apart.

Place your hands firmly on their sacrum area with your fingers facing out to the sides. Your wrists are centered in the middle of their sacrum.

Keep your arms straight and gently press down onto their sacrum using your body weight. This is a deep pose, so you may not need to apply too much pressure.

Maintain equal pressure on their inhalation and exhalation.

Maintain the assistance for as long as you feel is appropriate.

Release your hands and back away as they return to a seated position.

Perform the assist on the other side.

Yoga Prop Suggestions

Have them rest their head on a pillow or block.

Have them put a pillow or blanket under the hip of their bent leg.

What You Might Say (to help the process)

"Breathe deeply into your hips and lower back," "Keep your hips squared," "Soften your shoulders."

"I've lost my mind…thanks to yoga."
–John Feddersen, Devalila YogaTeacher

Pigeon Preparation—Option 2 Leg Pull

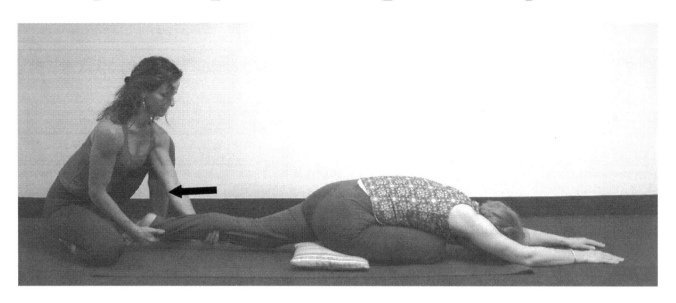

"Life is not a fixed point, but a never ending flow of creation. Dare to open yourself to the power within and create the life you were meant to have."
–Elizabeth Gill, Devalila Yoga Teacher

Assisting Steps for Pigeon Preparation Pose
(Leg Pull)

Kneel in the catcher's position close to their back foot.

Place one of your hands under their ankle and the other under the upper shin.

Lift their leg slightly and pull it toward you with a moderate force.

Maintain the assistance for as long as you feel is appropriate.

Release your hands, stand up, and back away as they return to a seated position.

Perform the assist on the other side.

Yoga Prop Suggestions

Have them rest their head on a pillow or block.

Have them put a pillow or blanket under the hip of their bent leg.

What You Might Say (to help the process)

"Let your hips melt toward the floor," "Keep your hips squared," "Relax your shoulders."

"Yoga allows you to turn off the noise and really hear the truth."
–Lyn Vencus, Yoga Student

Pigeon Preparation—Option 3
Diagonal Press

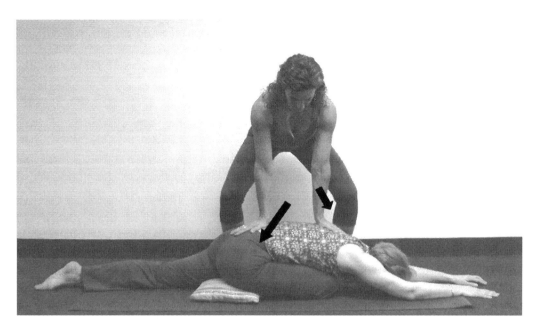

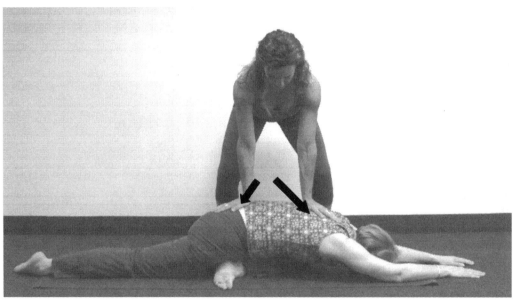

Assisting Steps for Pigeon Preparation Pose (Diagonal Press)

Stand with bent knees close to one side of the person's torso with your feet about hip width apart.

Place one of your hands on one side of their sacrum/upper buttocks and the other hand on the "mound" near their lower scapula blade. Your fingers are facing away from their spine.

While keeping your arms straight, gradually apply pressure onto their sacrum and shoulder using your body weight.

As you press down, aim your hands away from each other to give a diagonal stretch across their back. This is a deep pose, so you may not need to apply much pressure.

Change your hand position to the other shoulder and the other hip, and apply the same type of pressure described above.

Maintain the assistance for as long as you feel is appropriate. Lighten the pressure on their inhalation without losing contact with their body.

Release your hands and back away as they return to a seated position.

Have them switch legs and perform the assist on the other side.

Yoga Prop Suggestions

Have them put a pillow or blanket under the hip of the bent leg.

What You Might Say (to help the process)

"Breathe deeply into hips and lower back," "Keep your hips squared," "Relax your shoulders."

Reclining Knee to Chest

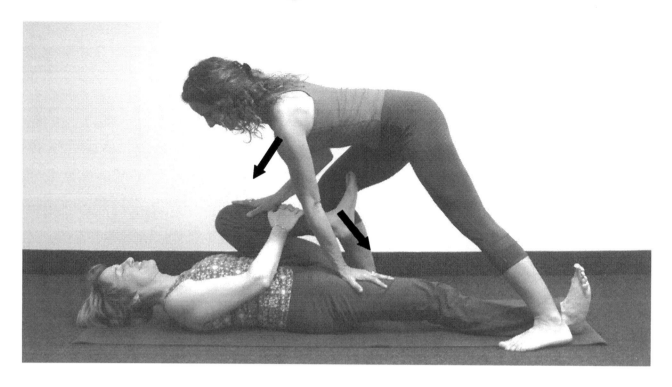

"There is nothing worse than a half-hearted assist. Don't rush. Take an extra breath and use conscious positioning to create a synergetic affect between you and the other person."
–John Feddersen, Devalila Yoga Teacher

Assisting Steps for Reclining Knee to Chest Pose

Straddle the person's outstretched leg in a standing squat position.

Step forward into a lunge position with your front leg near their bent leg.

Place one of your hands on the knee or shin of their bent leg (your fingers facing their face), and your other hand on the largest part of the thigh of their lower leg (your fingers facing their foot).

On their exhalation gradually apply equal pressure on both their legs, but in the opposite direction.

Maintain the assistance for as long as you feel is appropriate. Lighten the pressure on their inhalation.

Release your hands, stand up, and back away as they release their bent leg.

Perform the assist on the other side.

Yoga Prop Suggestions

None

What You Might Say (to help the process)

"Draw your hip toward your chest," "Keep your neck and shoulders relaxed," "Reach your outstretched leg toward the floor."

"Assists are just as organic and innate as the postures themselves and have to be nurtured and explored just the same." —Kelly Smith, Yoga Teacher, Pilates Teacher

Reclining Both Knees to Chest

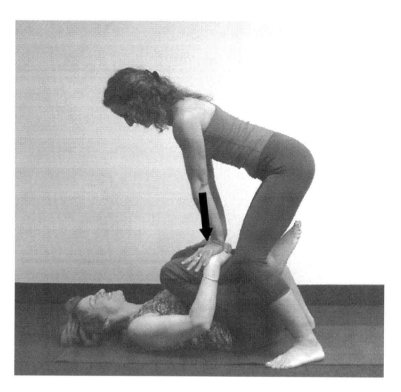

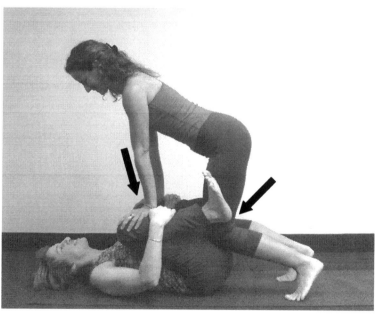

Assisting Steps for Reclining Both Knees to Chest Pose

Straddle the person's hips in a standing squat position.

Place your hands below their knees or on their shins (your fingers facing their face).

For a deeper stretch, you can separate their legs and press your knees into their hamstrings just above their sit bones (as in the bottom photo). Use the balls of your feet for balance in this variation.

On their exhalation, gradually apply pressure on both their knees using your body weight.

Maintain the assistance for as long as you feel is appropriate.

Release your hands, stand up, and back away as they return to a seated position.

~~~~~~

Yoga Prop Suggestions

None

What You Might Say (to help the process)

"Press your tail bone toward the floor," "Keep your neck and shoulders relaxed," "Draw your navel toward the floor on your exhalation."

"True peace is the knowledge that regardless of life's circumstances, all is eternally well."
—Elizabeth Gill, Devalila Yoga Teacher

Reclining Straight Leg Stretch

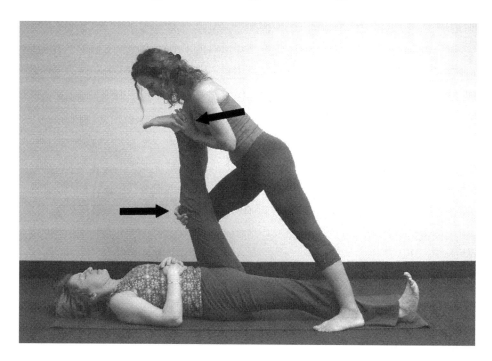

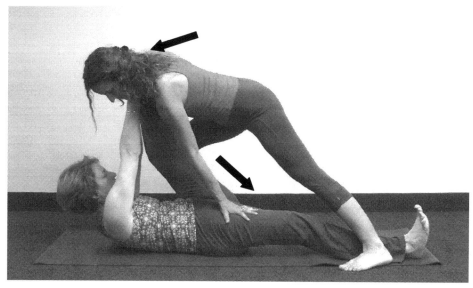

Assisting Steps for Reclining
Straight Leg Stretch Pose

Straddle the person's extended leg in a standing squat position.

Step forward into a lunge position with your front leg near their raised leg.

Place one of your hands on the knee of their raised leg and the other hand on their heel/ankle.

On their exhalation, slowly press their heel toward their head and keep their knee straight with your other hand (as in the top photo).

For a deeper stretch, you can have them reach up and pull on their leg as you simultaneously press the lower thigh toward the floor (as in the bottom photo).

Maintain the assistance for as long as you feel is appropriate.

Release your hands, stand up, and back away as they release their leg back to the floor.

Perform the assist on the other side.

Yoga Prop Suggestions

Have them wrap a yoga tie around the foot of their raised leg and draw it toward their torso.

What You Might Say (to help the process)

"Breathe deeply into hips and lower back," "Keep your neck and shoulders relaxed," "Reach your outstretched leg toward the floor."

Arm and Abdominal Strength Postures

The arm and abdominal strength poses are generally held for a shorter length of time. In some of these poses, the person is required to balance with limited contact with the floor, so assisting them can lessen feelings of doubt and instability that may arise. Since our arms are obviously occupied in these postures, it helps to have another set of arms to provide support! In this chapter I selected poses that demand even more arm and abdominal strength than other yoga poses. Here are some points to remember when assisting someone in the arm and abdominal strength poses:

- Check for alignment between their wrist, elbow, and shoulder when their arms are in a straight position.

- Don't lift them up so much that they are hardly working in the pose, or that they fall over.

- Don't lift them so much that you create a strain or misalignment in their lower back.

- Have them use yoga blocks under their hands.

- Ensure that their entire hand is in contact with the ground (there are exceptions when yoga blocks are used).

Note: All the postures in the following section should be performed for at least 20-30 seconds, but can be held for a bit longer depending on the needs of the student.

High Plank to Low Plank

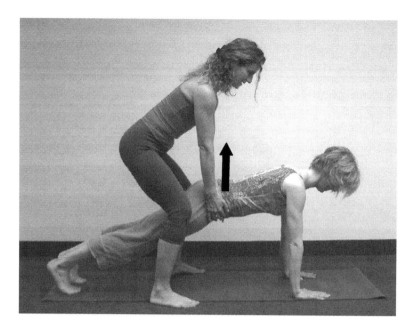

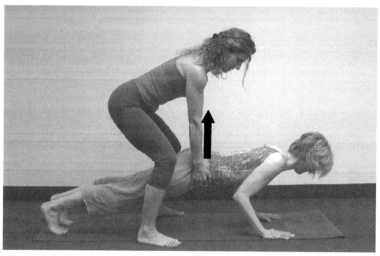

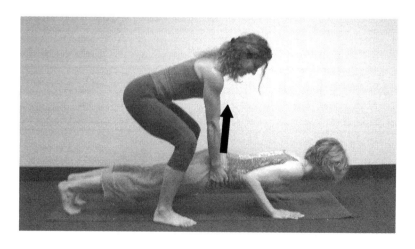

Assisting Steps for High Plank to Low Plank Pose

Straddle the person's upper legs in a standing squat position.

Use your hands to lift or lower their hips so that they are aligned with their shoulders and torso. Their lower back should be in a neutral position.

As they lower into low plank pose (as in the bottom photos) bend your knees and continue supporting their hips with your hands.

Visually, check to see that their elbows are near their rib cage, and that their upper arms are parallel to the floor (as in the bottom photo). If you see a misalignment, verbally instruct them to adjust their body while you are supporting their hips.

When they are established in low plank pose, release your hands and let them balance in the pose.

Stand up and back away as they lower to the floor.

Yoga Prop Suggestions

Have them place their hands on yoga blocks for extra lift.

What You Might Say (to help the process)

"Firm your buttocks and abdominal muscles as you lower to the floor," "Keep your neck long," "Hug your arms toward your rib cage," "Reach through your heels."

"Your external life is an exact reflection of your internal circumstances. If you want to see a change in your world, be the change." –Elizabeth Gill, Devalila Yoga Teacher

Side Plank

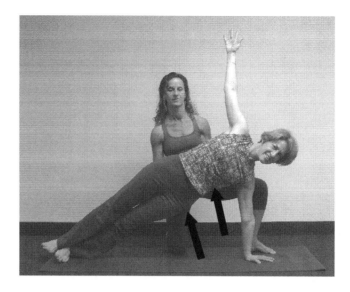

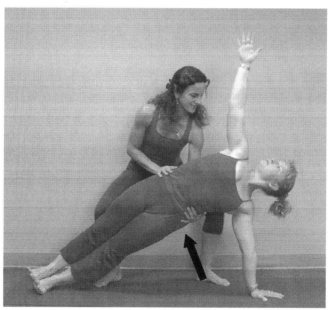

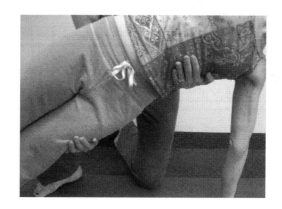

Assisting Steps in Side Plank Pose

Stand behind the person's torso and hips in a standing squat position (as in the bottom photos), or kneel in the catcher's position (as in the top photo).

Place one of your palms under their thigh area and the other under the rib cage area.

Use your hands to lift (or lower) their hips so that they are aligned with their shoulders and torso. Their lower back should be in a neutral position.

Visually, check their shoulder, elbow, and wrist alignment. If you see a misalignment, verbally instruct them to release the pose and adjust their arm position.

Maintain the assistance for as long as you feel is appropriate.

When they are established in side plank pose, release your hands and let them balance on their own.

Stand up and back away as they lower to the floor.

Yoga Prop Suggestions

Have them place their bottom hand on a yoga block for extra lift.

What You Might Say (to help the process)

"Squeeze your legs together," "Tuck your tailbone," "Lift your waist away from the floor," "Open your chest."

Upward Plank—Option 1
Support from Underneath

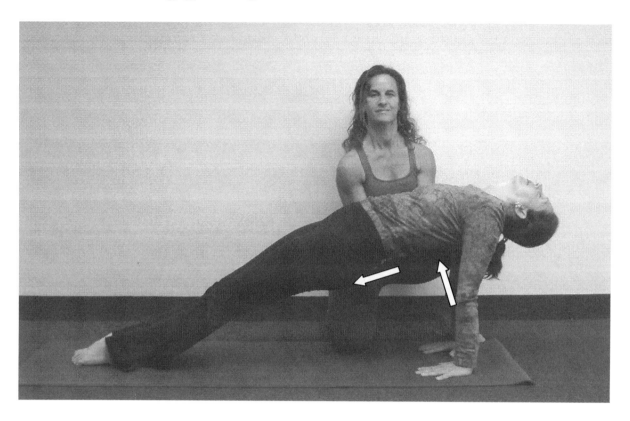

"My yoga practice has benefited every aspect of my life. By opening up and focusing on my breathing I become centered, let go of "stuff", and flow with the beauty of the moment."
–Lyn Vencus, Yoga Student

Assisting Steps for Upward Plank Pose
(Support from Underneath)

Kneel next to the person's torso and hips in the catcher's position.

Put one of your palms under their back between the scapula blades, and the other under the sacrum area.

Use your hands to lift their back and hips into the pose.

Tuck the pelvis slightly downward toward the tailbone as you lift upward.

Visually, check their shoulder, elbow, and wrist alignment. If you see a misalignment, verbally instruct them to release the pose and adjust their arm position.

Maintain the assistance for as long as you feel is appropriate.

When they are established in upward plank pose, release your hands and let them balance on their own.

Stand up and back away as they lower to the floor.

Yoga Prop Suggestions

Have them place their hands on yoga blocks.

What You Might Say (to help the process)

"Squeeze your inner legs and feet together," "Tuck your tailbone and firm your buttocks," "Actively point your toes toward the floor," "Breathe deeply into your chest."

Upward Plank—Option 2
Lift from Above

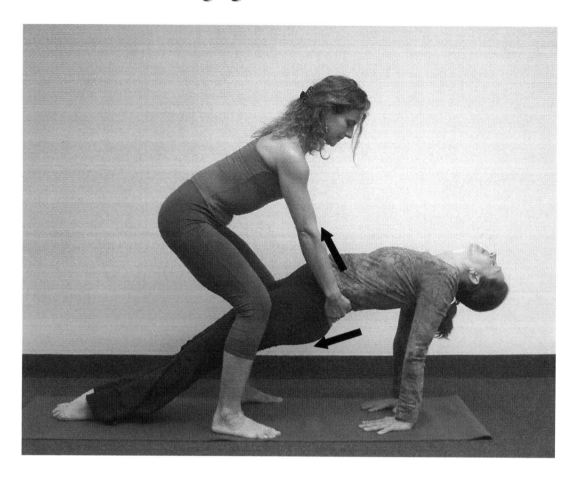

"Good yoga teachers are guides to a deeper experience that can be tapped into long after you leave the studio."
-Lyn Vencus, Yoga Student

Assisting Steps for Upward Plank Pose
(Lift from Above)

Straddle the person's upper legs in a standing squat position.

Use your hands to lift their hips so that they are aligned with their shoulders and torso.

Tuck the pelvis under as you lift the hips.

Visually, check their shoulder, elbow, and wrist alignment. If you see a misalignment, verbally instruct them to release the pose and adjust their arm position.

Maintain the assistance for as long as you feel is appropriate.

When they are established in upward plank pose, release your hands and let them balance on their own.

Stand up and back away as they lower to the floor.

Yoga Prop Suggestions

Have them place their hands on yoga blocks for extra lift.

What You Might Say (to help the process)

"Firm your buttocks and tuck your tailbone," "Open your chest toward the sky" "Engage your legs."

Crow

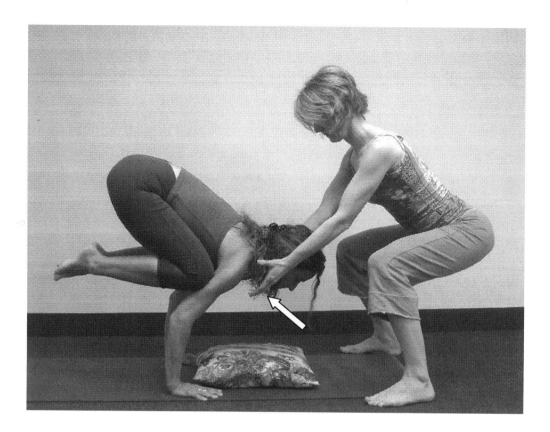

"I love being assisted in the postures and receiving personal attention. Yet sometimes in anticipation of the teacher's attention, I lose my concentration and fail to surrender to, or cooperate with, the instructor's assistance."
—John Feddersen, Yoga Teacher

Assisting Steps for Crow Pose

Stand in front of the person's shoulders in a deep standing squat position.

Place your hands just under their shoulders or collar bone without touching them.

As they lean forward into crow pose, be ready to catch them with your hands if they fall.

Visually, make sure that their hands are positioned under their shoulders and that they are gazing forward.

When they are established in crow pose, move your hands and let them balance on their own.

Stand up and back away as they lower their feet to the floor.

Yoga Prop Suggestions

Place a pillow under their face to soften a possible fall forward.

Have them place their hands on yoga blocks for extra lift.

What You Might Say (to help the process)

"Really engage your abdominal muscles," "Keep your gaze forward," "Draw your feet toward your buttocks," "Let your body weight come forward as you lift your feet."

Side Crow

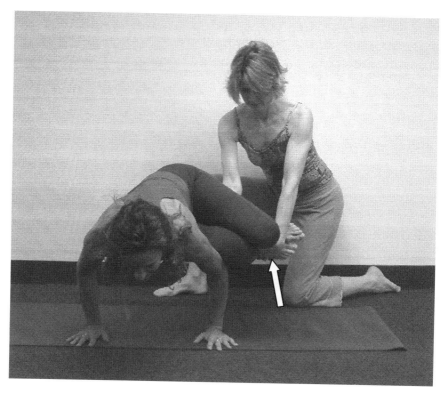

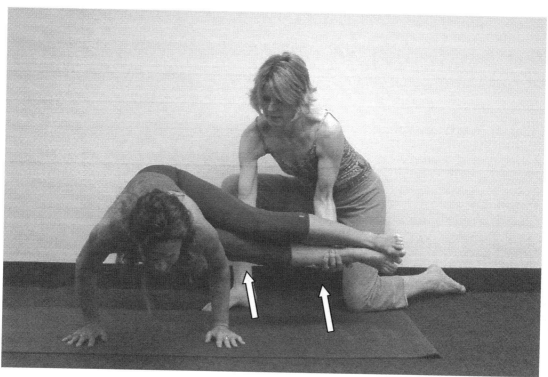

144

Assisting Steps for Side Crow Pose

Kneel in back of the person's legs in a catcher's position.

As their legs lift into side crow pose (as in the top photo), place your hands under or around their ankles and give them a slight lift.

If their legs are extending into full side crow pose (as in bottom photo), place your hands under knee and shin area and give them a slight lift.

Don't lift their legs too much or they may fall forward.

When they are established in side crow pose, release your hands and let them balance on their own.

Stand up and back away as they lower their feet to the floor.

Yoga Prop Suggestions

Place a pillow under their face to soften a possible fall forward.

Have them place their hands on yoga blocks for extra lift.

What You Might Say (to help the process)

"Really engage your abdominal muscles," "Keep your gaze forward," "Squeeze your legs together," "Let your chest lean forward as you lift your feet."

"The challenging postures remind us to have fun, stay focused, and let go of attachment to the results of our efforts." –Stephanie Pappas, Devalila Yoga Teacher and Trainer

Boat

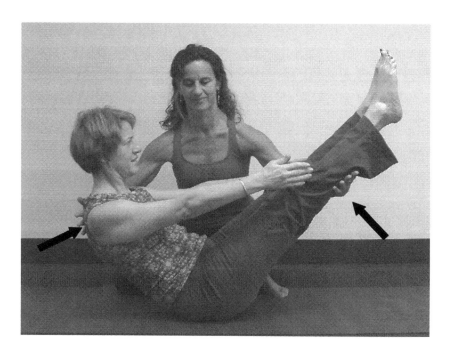

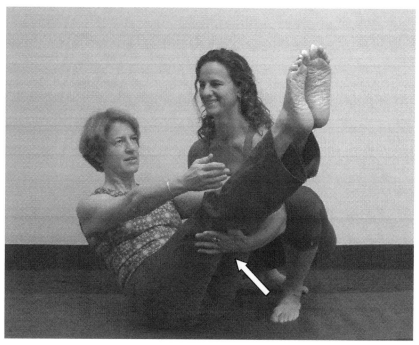

146

Assisting Steps for Boat Pose

Kneel to the side of the person's body in a catcher's position.

As their legs and torso lift into boat pose, place one of your hands under their calves and the other under their upper back.

Apply a gradual and equal lift to both the legs and back as if you were closing a book. Too much lift may tip them over in one direction or the other.

Maintain the assistance for as long as you feel is appropriate.

When they are established in boat pose, release your hands and let them balance on their own.

Stand up and back away as they lower their feet to the floor.

Yoga Prop Suggestions

Have them sit on a flat blanket as a cushion for their hips.

What You Might Say (to help the process)

"Bring your navel toward your spine," "Gaze toward your feet," "Squeeze your thighs together," "Lift your chest."

> "Now matter how I am feeling before class starts I feel better after."
> —Donna E. Poler, Devalila Yoga Student

Cow Face Arm Stretch

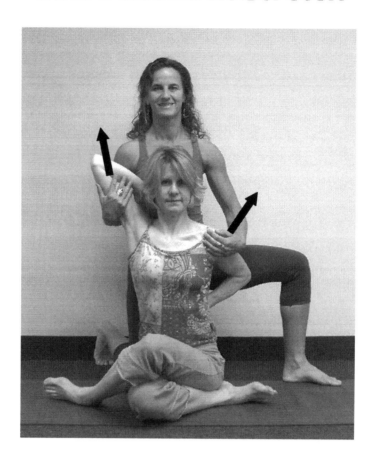

"Yoga shows me how to be stronger (emotionally or physically). I am grateful for what I have in my life."
–Tea Rodkey, Yoga Student

Assisting Steps for Cow Face Arm Stretch Pose

Kneel close to the person's back in the marriage proposal position with the front of your thigh aligned with their spine and to support their back.

Use one of your hands to hold the underside of their top arm and gradually draw it toward you.

Use your other hand to cup the deltoid of the bottom arm and gradually draw it toward you.

Maintain the assistance for as long as you feel is appropriate. Stay aware of their body and yours, and listen for their breath.

Release your hands and allow them to switch sides.

Perform the assist on the other side.

Yoga Prop Suggestions

Have them sit on the edge of a blanket or pillow.

What You Might Say (to help the process)

"Lengthen your spine, especially your low back," "Expand your chest," "Drop your shoulders away from your ears."

Twisting (Revolving) Postures

The revolving āsanas are challenging and invigorating. They demand flexibility, balance and strength. Twists are my favorite postures to assist and be assisted in. Here are some points to remember when assisting someone in the twisting poses in this section of the book:

- Anchor the base of the pose (usually their legs) before deeply twisting their torso.

- Have them use yoga blocks to help balance in certain standing twists.

- Use your whole hand and not just fingers when you twist them.

- Apply pressure in the same direction that the twist is moving.

- Remember to apply deeper pressure on their **exhalation**, and lighten the pressure on their **inhalation**.

Note: All the postures in the following section should be performed for at least 30 seconds, but can be held for much longer depending on the needs of the student.

Seated Twist (Beginner Version)

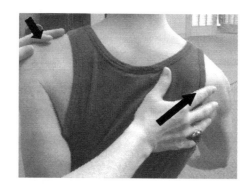

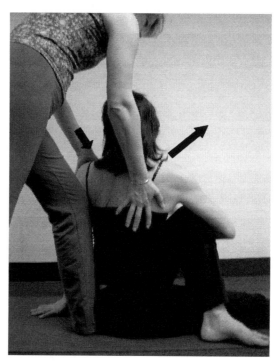

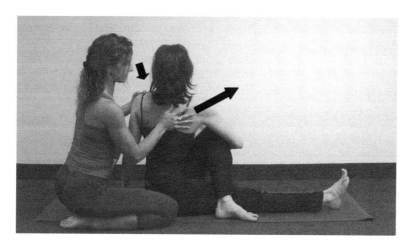

Assisting Steps for Seated Twist Pose
(Beginner Version)

Stand behind their back in a short standing lunge position (as in the middle photo) with your inner shin next to their spine.

You can also kneel facing their back in a catcher's position (as in the bottom photo).

Place one of your hands on the mound near their scapula blade. Press the shoulder in a forward direction (as in the top photo).

Simultaneously, cup your other hand around their front shoulder (deltoid area). Pull this shoulder toward you.

Twist their shoulders more on their exhalation and lighten the pressure on their inhalation. Keep your hands in contact with their body.

Release your hands and let them twist on their own before they return to a neutral seated position

Perform the assist on the other side.

Yoga Prop Suggestions

Have them sit on the edge of a blanket or pillow.

What You Might Say (to help the process)

"Twist deeper on your exhalation," "Get taller on your inhalation," "Lift up your lower back," "Keep your neck in alignment with the rest of your spine."

Seated Twist (Advanced Version)

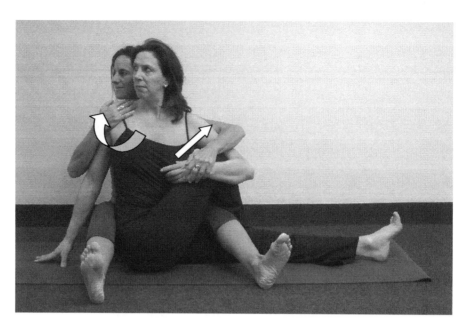

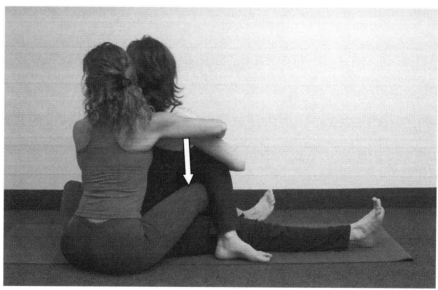

"There is yoga on the mat and off the mat. The real awakening happens when they become one." –Heidi Prewett, Devalila Yoga Teacher

Assisting Steps for Seated Twist Pose
(Advanced Version)

Sit behind their back with your legs spread wide.

Place one of your legs through the space made by their bent leg and press it down their thigh. Extend your other leg out near their low back.

Cup one of your hands around their shoulder that is leading the turn. Draw this shoulder toward you.

Simultaneously hug their other arm (the one that's holding their knee). Draw their arm and knee toward you.

Hug their whole upper body toward you. Twist their shoulders more on their exhalation.

Maintain the assistance for as long as you feel is appropriate.

Release your hands, slide your leg out of the hole, and let them twist on their own before returning to a neutral seated position.

Perform the assist on the other side.

Yoga Prop Suggestions

Have them sit on the edge of a folded blanket or pillow.

What You Might Say (to help the process)

"Twist deeply from your navel up to your neck," "Keep your sit bones on the floor," "Open your chest more as you twist."

Chair Twist

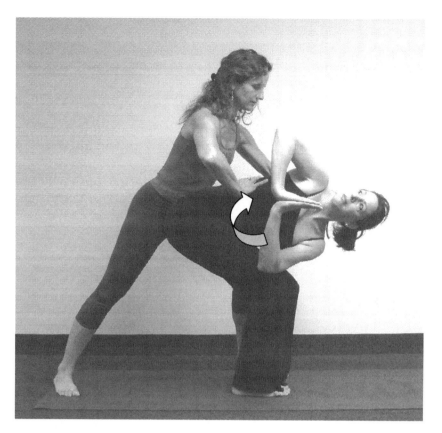

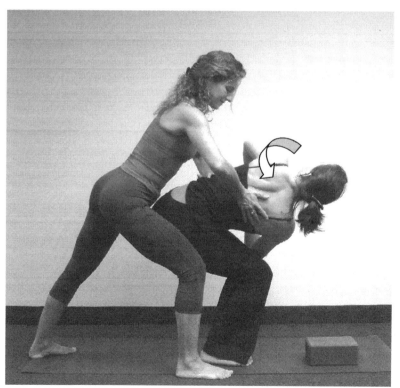

Assisting Steps for Chair Twist Pose

Stand in a lunge position with your front leg touching their outer hips (on the opposite from which they are facing).

Place one of your hands on the mound near the lower part of their scapula blade. Press this shoulder in a downward direction.

Simultaneously place your other hand (fingers facing away from their navel) on their rib cage (the ribs that are facing the sky). Press the rib cage in the same direction as your other hand.

Twist their torso deeper on the exhalation as you stabilize your own legs.

Maintain the assistance for as long as you feel is appropriate.

Release your hands and then slowly back away as they return to mountain pose.

Perform the assist on the other side.

Yoga Prop Suggestions

None

What You Might Say (to help the process)

"Keep your knees together," "Twist deeper on your exhalation," "Open your chest toward the ceiling," "Press your bottom elbow into your outer thigh."

"If you want to learn yoga, teach it!"
–Heidi Prewett, Devalila Yoga Teacher

Revolving Extended Angle Pose

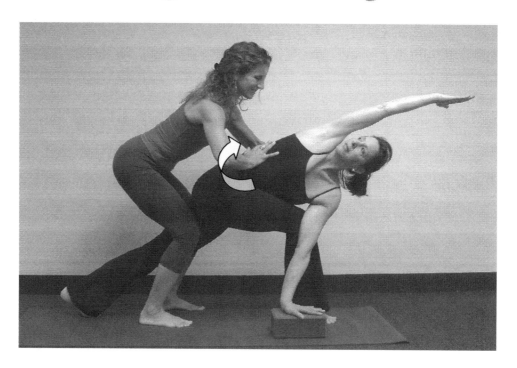

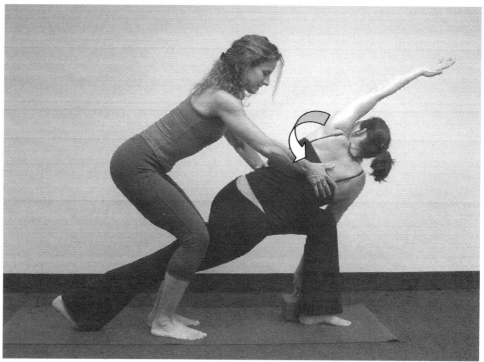

Assisting Steps for Revolving Extended Angle Pose

Straddle their back leg and bend your knees into the skier's squeeze position. Firmly squeeze their back leg with your legs.

Place one of your hands on the mound near the lower part of their scapula blade. Press this shoulder in a downward direction.

Simultaneously place your other hand (fingers facing away from their navel) on their rib cage (the ribs that are facing the sky). Press the rib cage in the same direction as your other hand.

Twist their torso deeper on their exhalations as you continue to stabilize their back leg.

Maintain the assistance for as long as you feel is appropriate.

Release your hands then slowly back away as they take they own weight. Allow them to return to forward fold or lunge pose before continuing with the other side.

Perform the assist on the other side.

Yoga Prop Suggestions

Have them put their lower hand on a yoga block for support (placed near the inside or outside of their front foot).

What You Might Say (to help the process)

"Keep your back leg strong," "Lift your back knee toward the sky," "Open your chest and armpit toward the ceiling," "Press your bottom arm against your outer knee for leverage in the twist," "Keep your hips parallel to the floor."

Revolving Triangle

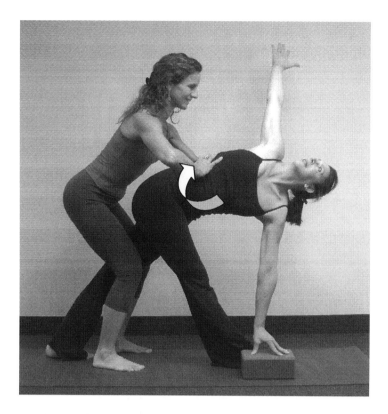

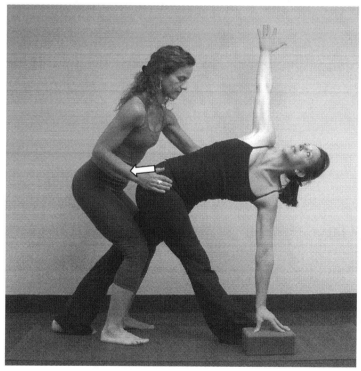

Assisting Steps for Revolving Triangle Pose

Straddle their back leg and bend your knees into the skier's squeeze position. Firmly squeeze their back leg with your legs.

Place one of your hands on the mound near the lower part of their scapula blade. Press this shoulder in a downward direction.

Simultaneously place your other hand (fingers facing away from their navel) on their rib cage (the ribs that are facing the sky). Press the rib cage in the same direction as your other hand.

You can use your hand (that is on the rib cage) to pull the hip of the front leg toward you. This action helps to square the hips (as in the bottom photo).

Twist their torso deeper on their exhalations as you continue to stabilize their back leg.

Maintain the assistance for as long as you feel is appropriate.

Release your hands then slowly back away as they take they own weight. Allow them to return to forward fold or mountain pose before continuing with the other side.

Perform the assist on the other side.

Yoga Prop Suggestions

Have them put their lower hand on a yoga block for support (placed near the inside or outside of their front foot).

What You Might Say (to help the process)

"Press firmly into both feet," "Square your hips," "Open your chest and armpit toward the ceiling," "Keep your neck in alignment with the rest of your spine."

Revolving Half Moon Two

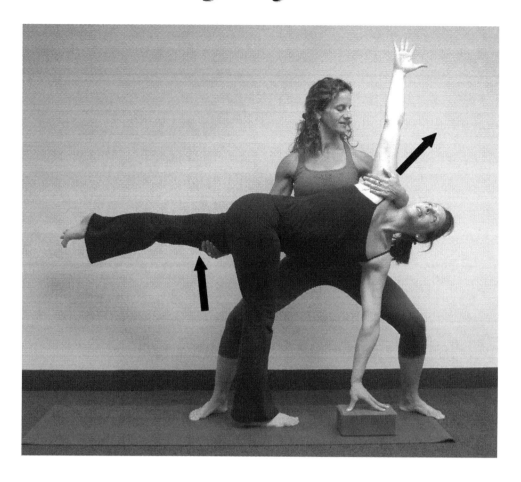

"Yoga is total transformation of mind and body; it connects you to the core of your heart and self-being." –Chanchal Arora, Devalila Yoga Teacher

Assisting Steps for Revolving Half Moon Two Pose

Stand behind the person with your belly or lightly touching their upper back. Make sure your stance is wide and very stable.

Use one of your hands (the one nearest their leg) to lift the thigh that is in the air.

Use your other hand (the one nearest their upper body) to cradle and lift the shoulder of the arm that is in the air.

Simultaneously draw their shoulder toward your body and lift their leg toward a horizontal position in the air.

Allow them lean their weight against you as if you were a wall.

Maintain the assistance for as long as you feel is appropriate.

Slowly release your hands, but remain standing there until they can balance on their own. Back away as they return to mountain pose.

Perform the assist on the other side.

Yoga Prop Suggestions

Have them place their lower hand on one or two yoga blocks.

Have them practice this pose against a wall.

What You Might Say (to help the process)

"Keep your hips square," "Energize your leg in the air," "Open your chest and armpit toward the sky," "If you feel off balance, look down."

Revolving Head to Knee Fold

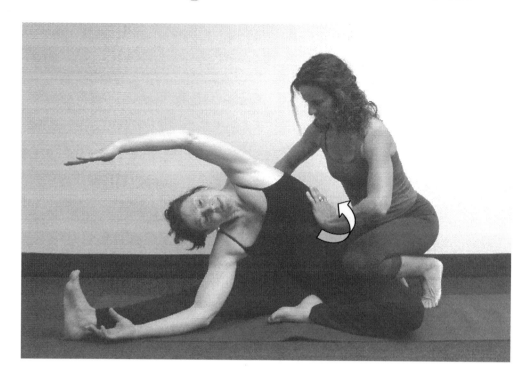

"Your students learn and appreciate more than you know."
–Carrie Colditz, Devalila Yoga Teacher

164

Assisting Steps for Revolving
Head to Knee Fold Pose

Kneel close to the person's back in the catcher's position with your upper shin on top of their bent leg (to anchor it down).

Place one of your hands on the mound near the lower part of their scapula blade. Press this shoulder in a downward direction.

Simultaneously place your other hand (fingers facing away from their navel) on their rib cage (the ribs that are facing the sky). Press the rib cage in the same direction as the other hand.

Apply a deeper pressure on their exhalation, and lighten the pressure on their inhalation (without losing contact).

Maintain the assistance for as long as you feel is appropriate.

Release your hands, stand up, and back away as they return to a seated position.

Perform the assist on the other side.

Yoga Prop Suggestions

Have them put pillows under their knees for support.

Have them press their outstretched foot into a wall for a deeper leg stretch.

What You Might Say (to help the process)

"Open your upper armpit toward the sky," "Reach your arm toward your outstretched leg," "Relax your head backward and look up."

Reclining Twist—Option 1 Diagonal Press

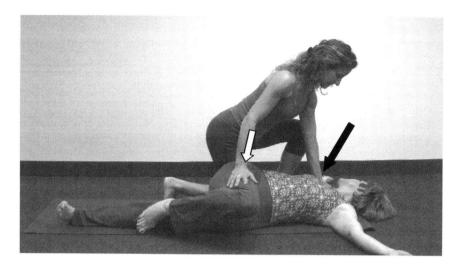

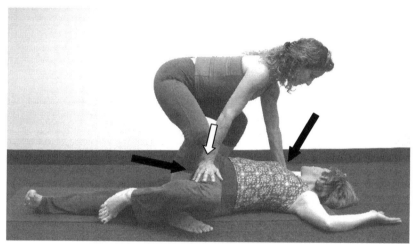

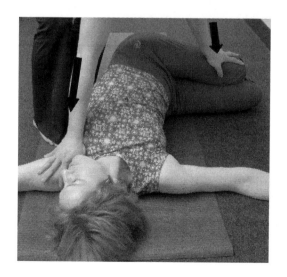

Assisting Steps for Reclining Twist Pose
(Diagonal Press)

Kneel close to the person's upper hip in the catcher's position (as in the top photo), or stand in a standing squat position (as in the bottom photos).

Place one of your hands on their front shoulder area (deltoid). Press this shoulder down toward the floor.

Simultaneously place your other hand (fingers facing away from their navel) on the side of their thigh, towards the middle. Press their leg(s) down toward the floor in the opposite direction from the shoulder.

Apply deeper pressure on their exhalation, and lighten the pressure on their inhalation (without losing contact).

Maintain the assistance for as long as you feel is appropriate.

Release your hands, stand up, and back away as they switch sides.

Perform the assist on the other side.

Yoga Prop Suggestions

Have them put a pillow under their bent knee(s) for support.

What You Might Say (to help the process)

"Relax your shoulders and back toward the floor," "Turn your head opposite direction from your knees," "Bring your knee closer to your ribs for a deeper stretch."

Reclining Twist—Option 2 Hip Pressure

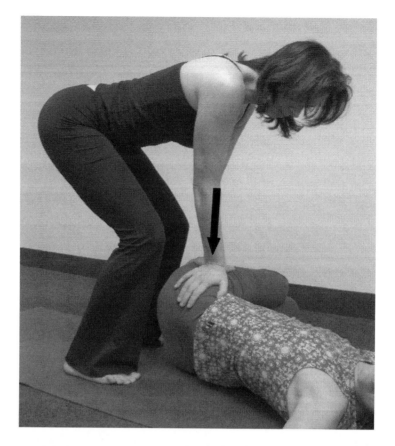

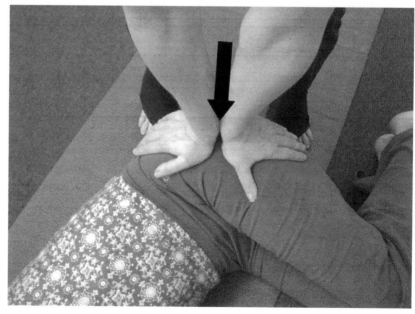

Assisting Steps for Reclining Twist Pose
(Hip Pressure)

Stand in a standing squat position next to the person's hips.

Place both of your hands on their hip bone area with your fingers facing away from each other.

Apply pressure directly downward on their hips.

Bend your knees and sink your weight sink down toward the ground. Keep your arms straight.

Maintain the assistance for as long as you feel is appropriate.

Release your hands, stand up, and back away as they switch sides.

Perform the assist on the other side.

Yoga Prop Suggestions

Have them put a pillow under their bent knee(s) for support.

What You Might Say (to help the process)

"Relax your shoulders and back toward the floor," "Bring your knee(s) closer to your ribs for a deeper stretch."

> "Getting out of the postures is as important as getting in."
> –Chanchal Arora, Devalila Yoga Teacher

Reclining Twist—Option 3 Arm Pull

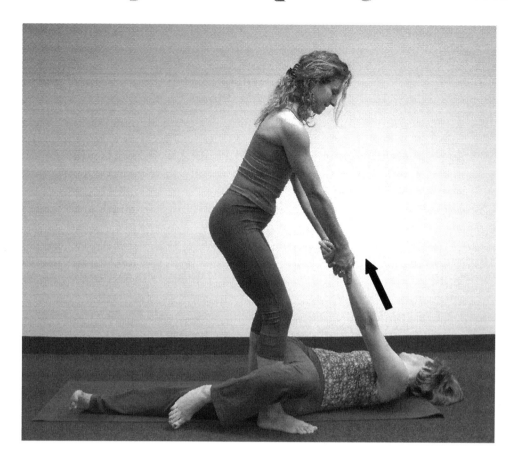

"When you first learn yoga you may think you know something—then you realize the practice is deeper and more mysterious than you thought. It just keeps changing!"
—Stephanie Pappas, Devalila Yoga Teacher and Trainer

Assisting Steps for Reclining Twist Pose (Arm Pull)

Stand in a standing squat position next to the person's hips. Put your leg (the one closest to their knee) into the crease of their bent knee and move it toward their torso.

Reach down and take hold of the wrist of their arm nearest to the bent knee.

Lift their arm and shoulder straight up until their shoulder comes off the floor (this action aligns their hips with their shoulders).

Place their arm back to the floor.

Now perform the reclining twist diagonal press.

Maintain the assistance for as long as you feel is appropriate.

Release your hands, stand up, and back away as they switch sides.

Perform the assist on the other side.

Yoga Prop Suggestions

Have them put a pillow under their bent knee for support.

What You Might Say (to help the process)

"Relax your shoulders and back toward the floor," "Breathe deeply into your lower back," "Soften your rib cage."

Back Bending Postures (Supine/Face-Up)

When you help someone with back bending postures that lift up, you lessen the burden of gravity on their body, and allow them to feel light, open and lengthened in their spine. Here are some points to remember when assisting someone in the supine back bending postures:

- Tuck their pelvis under when you are lifting them so that they don't over arch their low back.

- Remind the student to keep their legs and buttocks firm to help support their lower back.

- Remind the student to draw the navel inward to help support their lower back.

- Remind them not to jut their rib cage out of alignment with their hips.

Note: All the postures in the following section should be performed for at least 30 seconds, but can be held for much longer depending on the needs of the student.

Table Top—Option 1
Support from Underneath

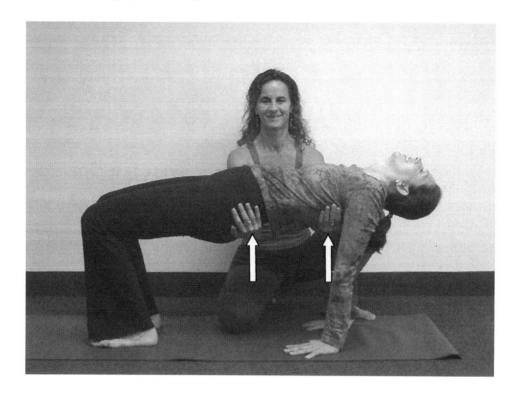

Assisting Steps for Table Top Pose
(Support From Underneath)

Kneel to the side of the person's body in a catcher's position.

As they lift into table top pose, place one of your arms (or hands) under their sacrum area and the other under their upper back with your fingers facing away from you.

Slowly lift up their back with both arms.

Maintain the assistance for as long as you feel is appropriate.

When they are established in table top pose, release your hands and let them hold the pose.

Stand up and back away as they lower their hips to the floor.

Yoga Prop Suggestions

Have them squeeze a yoga block between their knees to help engage their legs.

What You Might Say (to help the process)

"Engage your buttocks muscles," "Find a comfortable position for your neck," "Press down into your big toe joints," "Pull your navel toward your spine," "Lift and open your chest."

> "When my teacher touches me....I just melt."
> –Anonymous, Devalila Yoga Teacher, PA

Table Top—Option 2
Pelvic Lift from Above

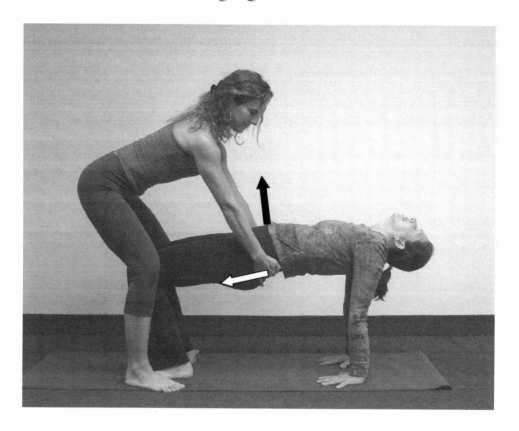

"When my teacher comes around to gently guide me into the correct position, I realize what the pose is supposed to feel like, and I can finally understand the relationship between the breath and the pose."
–Laurel Collins, Devalila Yoga Student

Assisting Steps for Table Top Pose
(Pelvic Lift from Above)

Straddle the person's knees in a standing squat position and apply a gentle pressure inward on their knees with your legs.

As they lift into table top pose, place your hands under their sacrum area with your fingers facing each other.

Lean your weight backward as if you were sitting into a chair and lift their back while you simultaneously tilt their pelvis under.

Maintain the assistance for as long as you feel is appropriate.

When they are established in table top pose, release your hands and let them hold the pose.

Stand up and back away as they lower hips to the floor.

Yoga Prop Suggestions

Have them squeeze a yoga block between their knees to help engage their legs.

What You Might Say (to help the process)

"Point your feet directly forward, or even a little pigeon-toed," "Firm your leg muscles," "Pull your navel toward your spine," "Lift and open your chest."

"We come into the world alone, but we also leave this world alone too. Just be okay with yourself." –Barbara Kulasinski, Photographer, Yoga Student

Bridge Formation

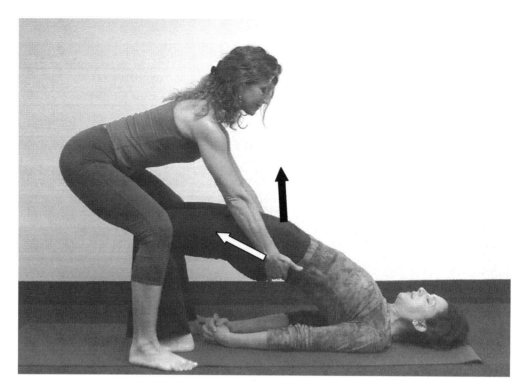

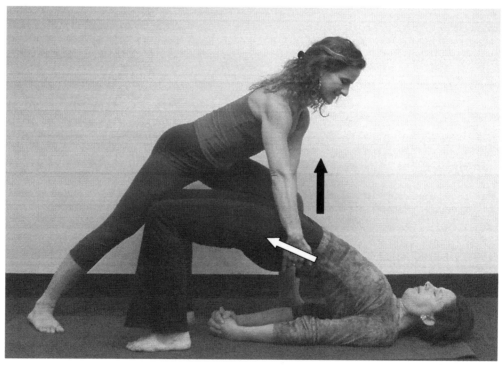

Assisting Steps for Bridge Formation Pose

Straddle the person's knees in a standing squat position and apply a gentle pressure inward on their knees with your legs (as in the top photo).

If the person is taller than you are, stand in a lunge position with your front foot alongside their hip area (as in the bottom photo).

As they lift up into bridge formation pose, place your hands under their sacrum area with your fingers facing each other.

Lean your weight backwards, and lift up their back with both of your hands. Simultaneously pull their hips toward you to help them lengthen their low back.

Maintain the assistance for as long as you feel is appropriate.

When they are established in the pose, release your hands and let them hold the pose.

Stand up and back away as they lower their hips to the floor.

Yoga Prop Suggestions

Have them squeeze a yoga block between their knees to help engage their legs.

Place a flat folded blanket under their shoulders to create space under the cervical spine.

What You Might Say (to help the process)

"Push into your feet," "Firm your buttocks muscles," "Shimmy your shoulders under your body," "Draw your navel toward your spine," "Breathe deeply and expand your chest."

Camel—Option 1 Chest Lift

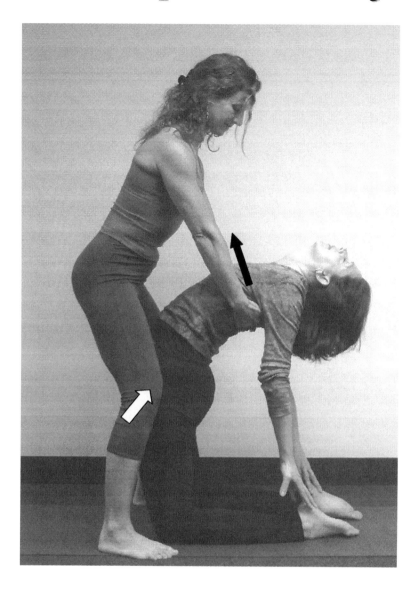

"Yoga inspires me to be me."
-Tea Rodkey, Yoga Student

Assisting Steps for Camel Pose (Chest Lift)

Straddle the person's hips in a standing squat position and apply a gentle pressure inward on their hips with your legs.

After they have arched back into camel pose, cradle their scapula bones with both hands (your finger tips are near their spine).

Lift their upper back with both hands, and at the same time stretch their scapula bones away from their spine.

Encourage them to breathe deeply into their chest and relax their shoulders.

Maintain the assistance for as long as you feel is appropriate.

When they are established in camel pose, release your hands and let them hold the pose.

You can lift them all the way up to a kneeling position when they are finished, or simply back away and allow them to return to a kneeling position on their own.

Yoga Prop Suggestions

Have them kneel on a flat folded blanket as a cushion.

What You Might Say (to help the process)

"Keep your thighs strong and moving forward," "Firm your buttocks muscles," "Expand your chest," "Breathe through your mouth if you need to."

Camel—Option 2 Foot Push

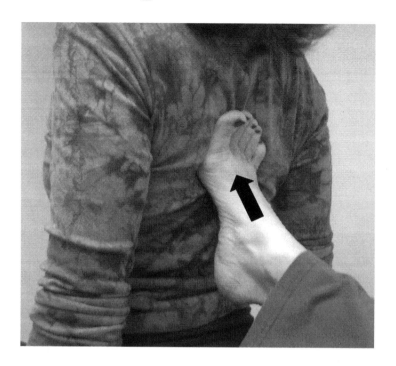

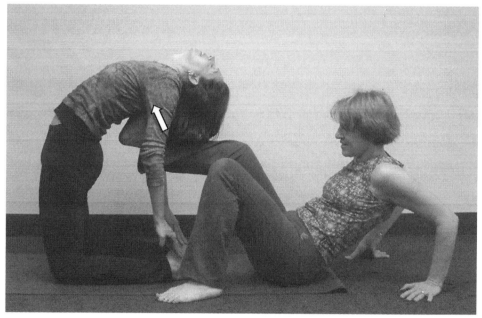

Assisting Steps for Camel Pose (Foot Push)

Sit behind the person's feet and put your hands behind you for support as you lean backwards.

Lift one of your feet in the air and place the ball of your foot between their scapula blades (as in the top photo).

After they arch backward into camel pose, carefully push the ball of your foot up into their back. Ask them for feedback about the placement of your foot and make any adjustments to the position.

As they breathe in the pose you can apply more pressure, but ensure that their hands stay in contact with their feet.

Maintain the assistance for as long as you feel is appropriate.

Release your foot and allow them to hold the pose on their own.

Sit up and back away as they return to an upright kneeling position.

Yoga Prop Suggestions

Have them place a flat folded blanket under their knees as a cushion.

What You Might Say (to help the process)

"Activate your thigh muscles," "Firm your buttocks muscles," "Let your shoulders relax toward the floor," "Relax your neck as much as possible."

"The inner silence that you can experience in yoga clears your perception. You emerge with a greater ability to listen and communicate from a space of love."
—Stephanie Pappas, Devalila Yoga Teacher and Trainer

Fish

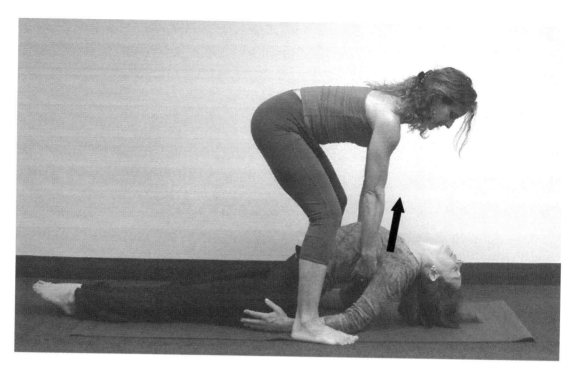

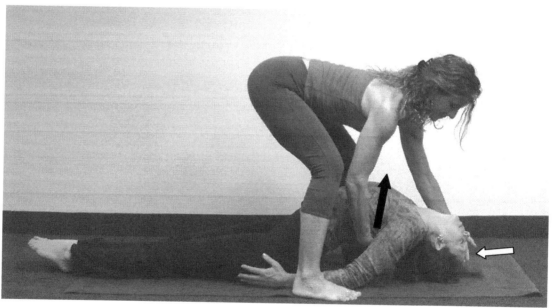

Assisting Steps for Fish Pose

Straddle the person's waist or hip area in a standing squat position.

Bend your knees and slide your hands under their upper back with your fingers near their spine.

Press into your legs, and slowly lift up their back with both hands. As you lift, also stretch the scapula blades away from their spine.

Encourage them to breathe deeply into their chest and relax their neck. Lift more on their inhalation.

When they are established in fish pose, remove one of your hands and gently tilt their forehead toward the floor and continue to lift with your other hand (as in the bottom photo).

Maintain the assistance for as long as you feel is appropriate. Stay aware of their body and yours, and listen for their breath.

Slowly slide your hands out from underneath their back, and move away as they lower themselves to the floor.

Yoga Prop Suggestions

Place a flat folded blanket or a pillow under the top of their head.

Place a pillow under their upper back.

Place a rolled up blanket under the length of their spine.

What You Might Say (to help the process)

"Press down into your elbows," "Relax your shoulders toward the floor," "Lift your chest."

Wheel—Option 1 Holding Teacher's Ankles

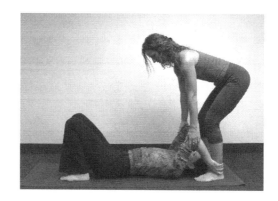

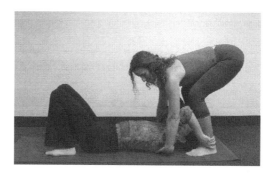

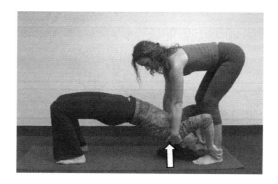

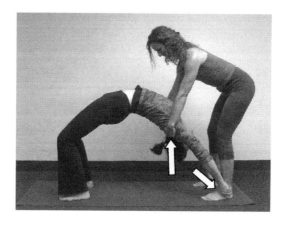

Assisting Steps for Wheel Pose
(Holding Teacher's Ankles)

Ask the student to get into the ready position for wheel pose (as in the top photo).

Stand about one foot (the distance may vary depending on their arm length) behind the person's shoulders in a standing squat position.

Instruct the student to hold firmly onto your ankles with their thumbs on your inner ankle. Their elbows are facing the sky and bent at about a 45 degree angle.

Bend down and reach your hands over their armpits and grab onto their scapula bones with your fingers facing their spine.

Lift their body off the floor with the strength of your legs

Instruct them to push their hands into your ankles.

As they lift further off the floor, support their shoulders with your hands.

Maintain the assistance for as long as you feel is appropriate. Stay aware of their body and yours, and listen for their breath.

To release the pose, tell them to bring their chin toward their chest as you bend your knees and lower them to the floor.

Yoga Prop Suggestions

Have them squeeze a yoga block between their knees to help engage their legs.

What You Might Say (to help the process)

"Tuck your tail bone under," "Push strongly into my ankles," "Lean your weight into your feet and legs," "Breathe deeply and expand your chest."

Wheel—Option 2 Two People Assisting

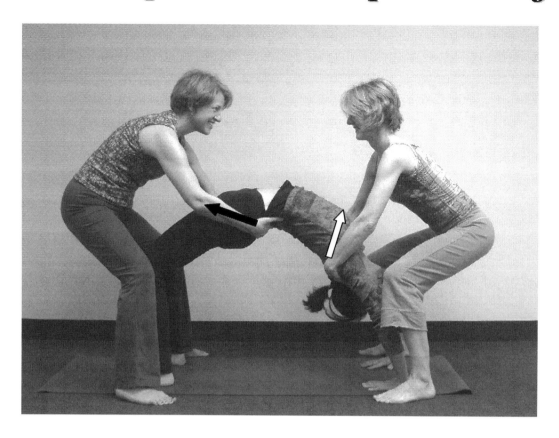

"Sometimes, no matter how carefully I describe what they should be doing or feeling, an assist is worth several thousand words."
—John Feist, Devalila Yoga Teacher

Assisting Steps for Wheel Pose
(Two People Assisting)

Allow the student to lift up into wheel pose on their own. Both assistants will then perform their parts simultaneously.

<u>Assistant 1</u> (on the left): Straddle the person's feet in a standing squat position, and if necessary, apply a gentle pressure inward on their knees with your legs.

Place your hands under their sacrum area with your fingers facing each other.

Lean your weight backwards, and pull their sacrum toward you to help lengthen their low back.

<u>Assistant 2</u> (on the right): Straddle the person's hands in a standing squat position.

Reach your hands over their armpits and grab onto their scapula blades with your fingers facing their spine.

Lift their body away from the floor using the force of your legs.

Maintain the assistance for as long as you feel is appropriate. Stay aware of their body and yours, and listen for their breath.

Both assistants guide the person back to the floor, release your hands and back away.

Yoga Prop Suggestions

Have them squeeze a yoga block between their knees to help engage their legs.

What You Might Say (to help the process)

"Point your feet directly forward, or a little pigeon-toed," "Press your weight into your legs and feet," "Drop your shoulders away from your ears," "Draw your navel toward your spine," "Breathe deeply and expand your chest."

Back Bending Postures (Prone/Face-Down)

Prone back bending postures require shoulder flexibility and back strength. Like the supine back bending postures, the person is working against gravity, but in the prone position there are more demands on the whole back and less on the legs. By assisting someone in the prone back bending postures you can really help them lift and open their chest. Here are some points to remember when assisting someone with the prone/face down back bending postures:

• Lift them gradually when you are taking them deeper into the back bend.

• Remind the person to keep their legs and buttocks firm, and draw their navel inward to afford safety to their lower back.

• Remind the person to drop their shoulders away from their ears and open the front of their chest.

• Encourage them to breathe fully into their chest and diaphragm.

Note: All the postures in the following section should be performed for at least 30 seconds, but can be held for much longer depending on the needs of the student.

Cat Stretch

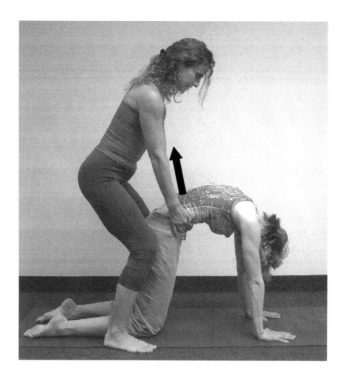

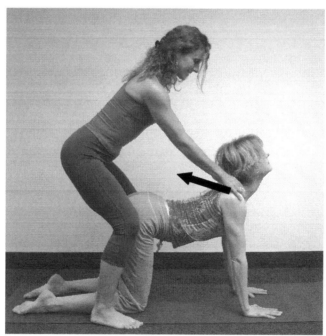

Assisting Steps for Cat Stretch Pose

Straddle the person's hips in a standing squat position.

As they flex their spine, use your hands to lift their waist and tilt their pelvis under (as in top photo).

As they extend their spine, use your hands to draw back their shoulders and promote chest expansion (as in bottom photo).

Repeat these two movements as they continue to contract and arch their back.

Maintain the assistance for as long as you feel is appropriate.

Stand up and back away as they return to a seated position.

Yoga Prop Suggestions

Have them kneel on a flat folded blanket as a knee cushion.

What You Might Say (to help the process)

"Exhale and tuck your tailbone under," "Inhale and open your chest," "Press into your hands," "Let your spine move smoothly and fluidly."

"My yoga teacher encourages me to do and be my best, while also asking that I be kind and gentle to myself."–Donna E. Poler, Devalila Yoga Student

Half Locust

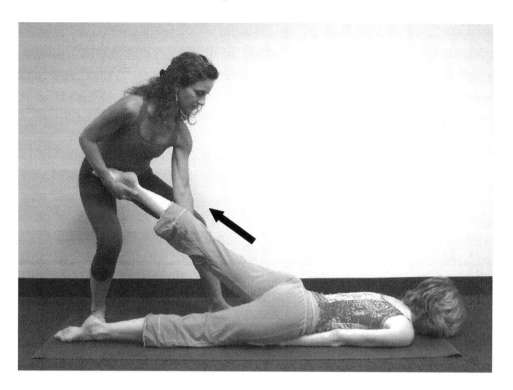

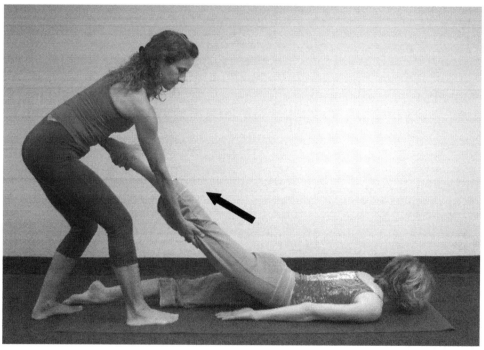

Assisting Steps for Half Locust Pose

Stand to one side of the person's feet in a standing squat position.

As they lift one of their legs into half locust pose, place one of your hands under their knee area and your other hand under their ankle.

Use your hands to lift their leg and pull it toward you.

Maintain the assistance for as long as you feel is appropriate.

Slowly bring their leg to the floor and switch sides.

Perform the assist on the other side.

Yoga Prop Suggestions

Have them lie on a flat folded blanket as a hip cushion.

What You Might Say (to help the process)

"Point your toes and extend through your legs," "Keep your upper body relaxed," "Engage your buttocks muscles."

"My teacher adeptly mixes deep spirituality with fun and a great workout for the body and mind."–Donna E. Poler, Devalila Yoga Student

Cobra

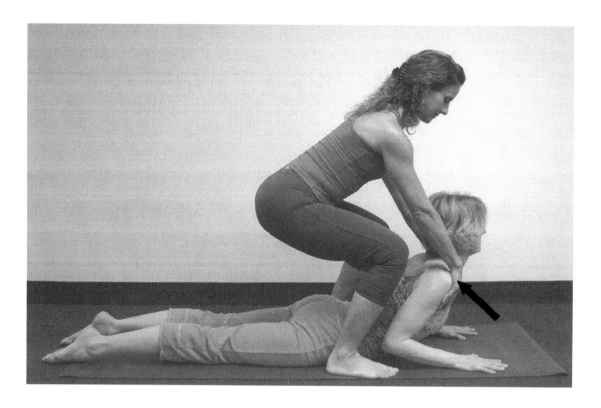

Assisting Steps for Cobra Pose

Straddle the person's hips in a standing squat position.

As they lift their spine into cobra pose, place your hands on the front of their shoulders and upper chest.

Use your hands to lift their body and draw back their shoulders.

Increase the lift on their inhalation.

Maintain the assistance for as long as you feel is appropriate.

Slowly release them back to the floor and step out of the straddle position.

Yoga Prop Suggestions

Have them lie on a flat folded blanket as a hip cushion.

What You Might Say (to help the process)

"Keep your buttocks and legs firm," "Drop your shoulders away from your ears," "Hug your elbows toward your rib cage," "Press into your hands."

> "A little touch goes a long way!" –Kerrie Anczarki, Devalila Yoga Teacher, Kids Yoga Teacher

Snake

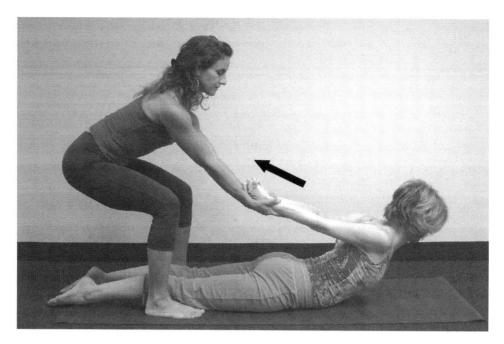

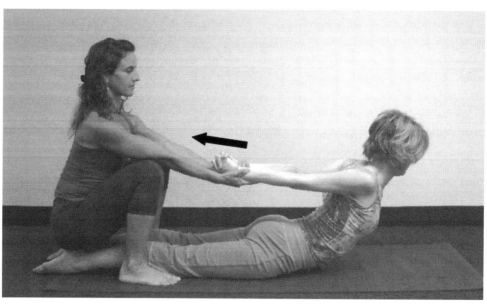

Assisting Steps for Snake Pose

Straddle the person's knees in a standing squat position.

As they lift their arms and back into snake pose, firmly hold onto their wrists or forearms.

Pull their arms toward you and sink your weight into your hips.

To take them even deeper into the pose, walk backward and sit down over their feet (as in the bottom photo).

Lift them more on their inhalation.

Maintain the assistance for as long as you feel is appropriate.

Slowly stand up and return them to the floor. Release your hands and step out of the straddle position.

~~~~~~

Yoga Prop Suggestions

Have them lie on a flat folded blanket as a hip cushion.

What You Might Say (to help the process)

"Keep your buttocks and legs firm," "Drop your shoulders away from your ears," "Expand your chest."

> "With my yoga instructor assisting me in the posture, and with the 'up and over' breathing sense in my posture, my yoga posture was able to become deeper and more enjoyable."
> –Carol Mauger, Yoga Teacher and Student

Upward Dog

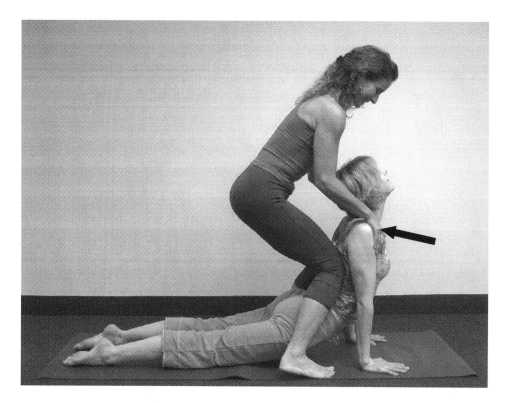

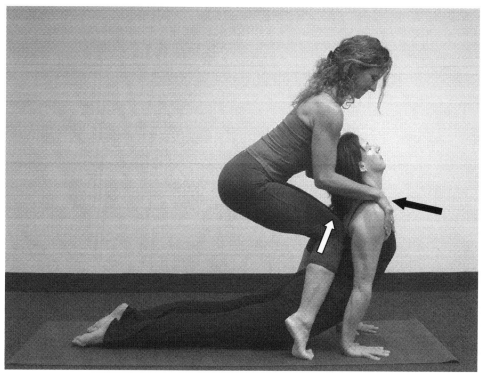

Assisting Steps for Upward Dog Pose

Straddle the person's hips in a standing squat position.

As they lift into upward dog pose, place your hands on the front of their shoulders and upper chest.

Use your hands to lift their body and draw their shoulders backward.

Lift them more on their inhalation.

To give them an extra stretch, rise up onto the balls of your feet, knock your knees inward, and press your knees into their upper back (if your knees can reach).

Pull their chest open as you push your knees into their back.

Maintain the assistance for as long as you feel is appropriate.

Release your knees, slowly lower them to the floor, and step out of the straddle position.

Yoga Prop Suggestions

Have them place their hands on yoga blocks for extra lift.

What You Might Say (to help the process)

"Keep your buttocks and legs firm," "Drop your shoulders away from your ears" "Pull your hips toward your wrists," "Lift your knees away from the floor."

Bow

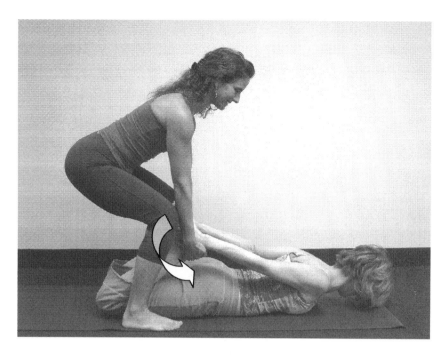

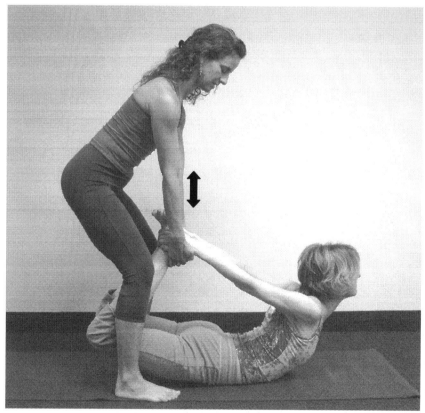

Assisting Steps for Bow Pose

Straddle the person's knees in a standing squat position.

As they lift into bow pose, reach your hands around the outside of their wrists and hold onto their heels (as in the top photo).

Keep your arms straight and use your leg strength to lift their body up (as in the bottom photo).

Lift them more on their inhalation.

Maintain the assistance for as long as you feel is appropriate.

Slowly release them back to the floor, release their heels, and step out of the straddle position.

Yoga Prop Suggestions

Have them lie on a flat folded blanket as a hip cushion.

What You Might Say (to help the process)

"Reach your feet toward the sky," "Press your feet backward away from your hips," "Breathe deeply into your chest and diaphragm."

> "Don't be shy to give your teacher or partner feedback—especially when you want them to change the level of pressure they are applying."
> —Stephanie Pappas, Devalila Yoga Teacher and Trainer

Inverted Postures

Inverted postures give us the opportunity to challenge our fears, turn our world upside down for awhile, and do something out of the ordinary with our bodies. Some people consider inversions to be the most beneficial of all yoga postures. It's extremely helpful and wise to assist someone when they are learning inversions. Here are some points to remember when assisting someone in inverted āsanas:

- Never force someone into a headstand. If you have to help them too much, it may mean that their alignment is off. If their alignment is off, you don't want them up in a headstand. They may be able to "float" into a headstand if their body is properly aligned (see pages on "floating" into a headstand).

- Encourage the person to take their time, breathe, and stay very aware of cues from the assistant when learning inverted postures.

- Give the person plenty of verbal guidance when learning to invert since they probably won't be able to see you, and they may get physically disoriented.

- Clear the practice area of objects and furniture.

- Perform inversions on a flat, stable surface.

- Offer folded blankets for under their shoulders in plow and shoulder stand postures.

- Check for adequate space between the wall and the person performing the pose (about 5-7 inches).

Note: All the postures in the following section should be performed for at least 20-30 seconds, but can be held for a shorter or longer duration depending on the needs of the student.

Plow—Option 1 Beginner Variation

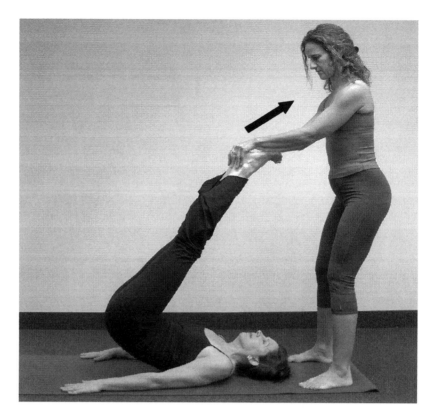

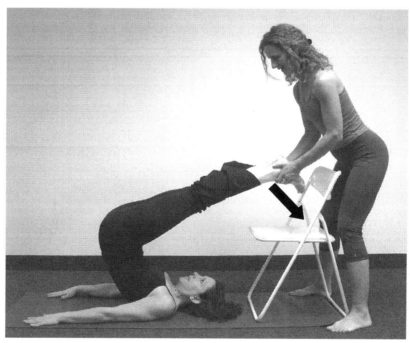

Assisting Steps for Plow Pose (Beginner Variation)

Stand about 1 foot behind the person's head.

As they lift their legs into plow pose, hold their heels and draw them toward you (as in the top photo).

While holding their heels, slowly walk backward and their hips will lift off the floor.

Instruct them to place their hands under their back or hips for balance.

Guide their feet toward the floor or toward a chair if they cannot touch the floor (as in the bottom photo).

Maintain the assistance until their feet touch something solid.

When they are established in the pose, release your hands and let them hold the pose.

You can now perform the pelvic lift adjustment described on the following pages.

Yoga Prop Suggestions

Have them place their feet on a chair, stool, or other yoga prop.

Have them place a flat folded blanket under their shoulders to create space under their cervical spine.

What You Might Say (to help the process)

"Let your knees bend if your hamstrings are tight," "Shimmy your shoulders under your body," "Support your back with your hands," "Relax your jaw and neck."

Plow—Option 2 Pelvic Lift

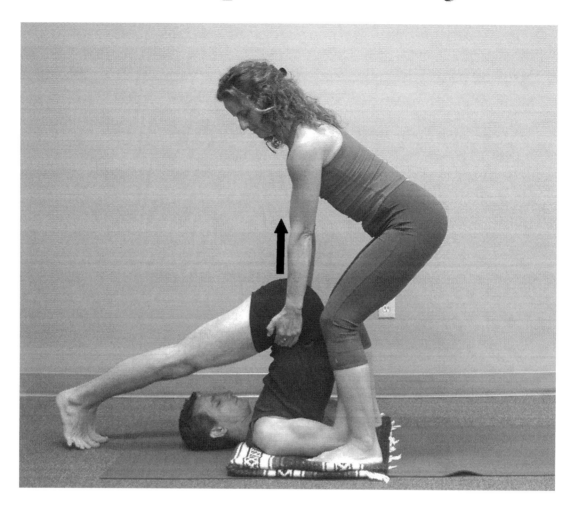

"The help of the teacher was very positive and reinforcing, and I have been able to give this sense to reinforcement and affirmation to others."
–Carol Mauger, Yoga Teacher and Student

Assisting Steps for Plow Pose (Pelvic Lift)

Stand close behind the person's back in a standing squat position.

Place your fingers in the crease made by their bent legs.

Using your leg strength, lift their hips straight up with both hands and let them to roll their shoulders under their body.

Maintain the assistance for as long as you feel is appropriate.

Release your hands and let them hold the pose.

Back away as they roll their spine back to the floor.

Yoga Prop Suggestions

Have them place their feet on a chair, stool or other yoga prop.

Have them place a flat folded blanket under their shoulders to create space under their cervical spine.

What You Might Say (to help the process)

"Move your tailbone away from your face," "Shimmy your shoulders under your body," "Lengthen your spine," "Breathe deeply into your upper back."

> "The assistor is able to learn first hand the abilities and limitations of the assisted. This knowledge makes it possible to provide recommendations for an individual's future practice."
> —Daniel Farrell, Devalila Yoga Teacher, Scientist

Shoulder Stand

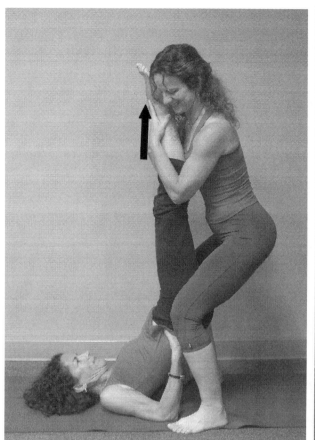
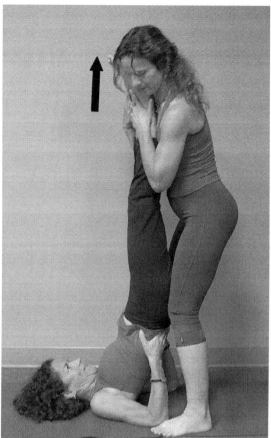
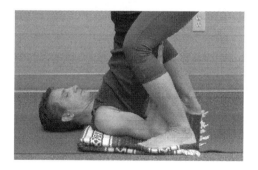

Assisting Steps for Shoulder Stand Pose

Stand close behind the person's back in a standing squat position with your feet near, or touching their elbows.

Place your hands and forearms around their shins.

Bend your knees and then gradually stand up straight as you simultaneously pull their legs toward the sky.

Instruct them to roll their shoulders under as you nudge their elbows in with your feet.

Assist them for as long as you feel is appropriate.

When they are established in the pose, release your hands and let them balance on their own.

Yoga Prop Suggestions

Have them place a flat folded blanket under their shoulders to create space under their cervical spine.

What You Might Say (to help the process)

"Reach your feet toward the sky," "Shimmy your shoulders under your body," "Engage the buttocks muscles," "Walk your hands up your back."

> "Possibly because of the number of ways assistance communicates (position, touch movement, real-time observation, sharing), awareness is focused and learning is rapid. It feels great and is reassuring." –Daniel Farrell, Devalila Yoga Teacher, Scientist

Forearm Stand

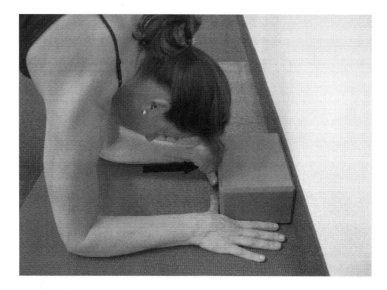

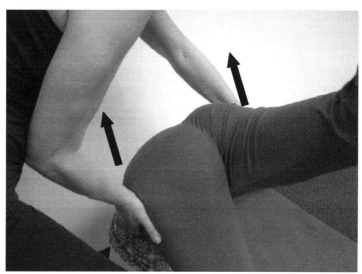

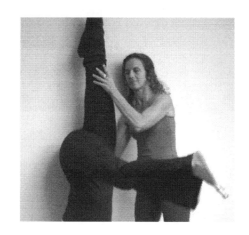

Assisting Steps for Forearm Stand Pose

Place a yoga block next to the wall.

Instruct them to press their thumbs on the front of the block, and their index fingers along the side of the block (as in the top photo).

Stand to one side of the person near their legs.

Place your hands in their thigh crease with your fingers facing each other (as in the middle photo).

Give their hips a gentle lift as they reach (or kick) their leading leg toward the wall (remember to stay out of the way of their leg!).

You can also press their leading leg toward the wall (as in the bottom photo) as they kick up.

When they are established in the pose, release your hands and let them balance on their own.

Now your can perform the fist squeeze as described later in this chapter.

Yoga Prop Suggestions

Have them perform this pose in front of a wall.

Have them press a yoga block into the wall with their hands.

What You Might Say (to help the process)

"Point your toes toward the sky," "Press your shoulders down away from your ears," "Gaze between your hands."

Handstand—Option 1 Kicking onto the Wall

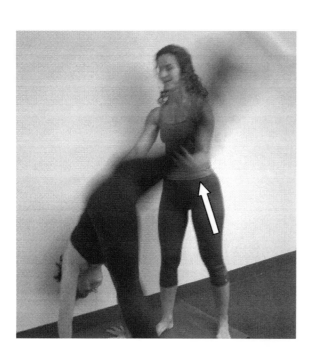

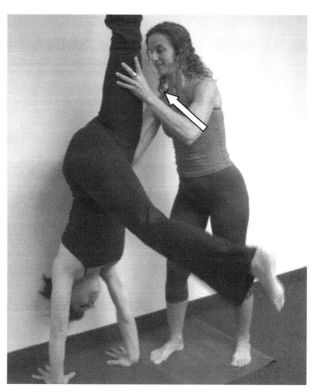

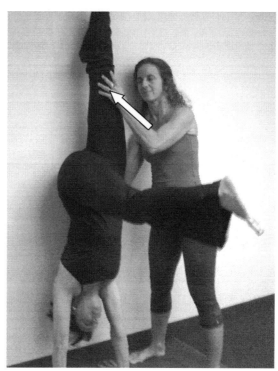

Assisting Steps for Handstand Pose
(Kicking onto the Wall)

Have them place their hands about 5-7 inches from the wall.

Stand to one side of the person near their legs (preferably the leg that will kick up first).

Place one hand one their low back for stability (optional).

Watch carefully as they prepare to kick their legs up—it can happen fast!

With your other hand(s), bring their kicking leg to the wall and then help the trailing leg toward the wall.

When both of their feet are touching the wall, release your hands and let them balance on their own.

Now you can perform the fist squeeze as described later in this section.

Yoga Prop Suggestions

Have them perform this pose in front of a wall.

What You Might Say (to help the process)

"Reach your toes toward the sky," "Keep your shoulders over your hands," "Squeeze your inner thighs together," "Firm your whole body."

"Inversions are so energizing! Let your teacher help you overcome your fears."
—Stephanie Pappas, Devalila Yoga Teacher and Trainer

Handstand—Option 2 Two People Spotting

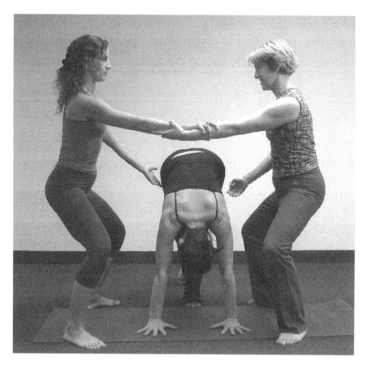

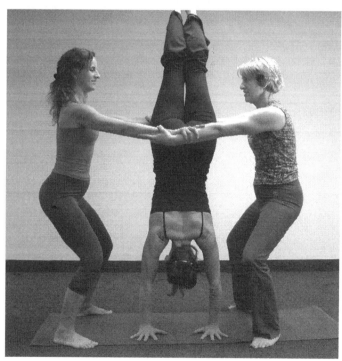

Assisting Steps for Handstand Pose
(Two People Spotting)

Two assistants will stand facing each other in standing squat positions.

Reach out toward each other with the same arm (the arm that is farthest away from the person) and hold each other's forearms.

Instruct the student to place their hands in the center of the floor between you (as in the top photo).

Watch carefully for the student's next move to kick their legs up.

When both of the student's legs are in the air, quickly reach out toward each other with your free arm and clasp each other's forearms. Enclose their legs between your arms.

Allow the student's legs or hips to rest against your arms, or vacillate between your arms as the find their balance.

When they are finished with the pose, release your hands, and allow them to return their feet to the floor.

Yoga Prop Suggestions

None

What You Might Say (to help the process)

"Point your toes a lot," "Pull your navel toward your spine," "Squeeze your inner thighs together," "Press your hands into the floor."

Headstand Preparation (Tripod)

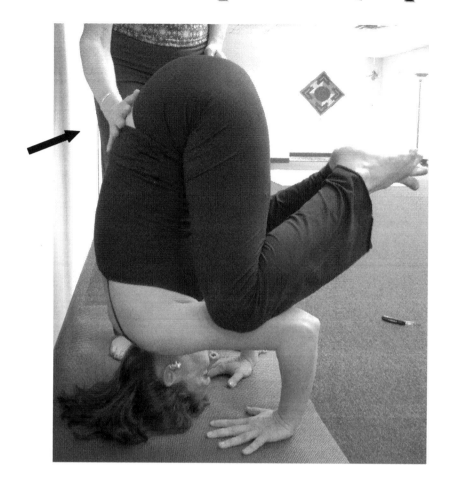

"You'll find some people will improve their breathing and better relax in a pose when you're very physically assisting."
–Carrie Colditz, Devalila Yoga Teacher

Assisting Steps for Headstand Preparation Pose (Tripod)

Stand or kneel on one side of the person near their shoulders.

Visually, assess their headstand set up alignment (see tips on "floating" into headstand) and verbally instruct them to make changes in their head or hand placement.

As they are in tripod position, place your hand on their sacrum and encourage them to tilt their pelvis back toward your hand.

Help them place their knees on their triceps.

Keep checking their alignment and give verbal feedback.

If their legs begin to "float" up, follow the instructions for headstand assisting.

Yoga Prop Suggestions

Have them perform this pose in front of a wall.

What You Might Say (to help the process)

"Bring your feet toward your hips," "Bring your hips over your shoulders," "Press your shoulders down," "Gaze forward to the floor in front of you."

"Yoga enables me to stretch in many areas of my life and to go with patience into places I have not been before."—Madonna Alvarez, Devalila Yoga Student

219

Headstand (Supported)

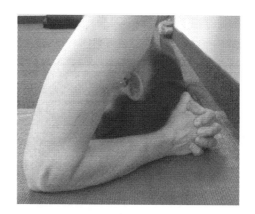

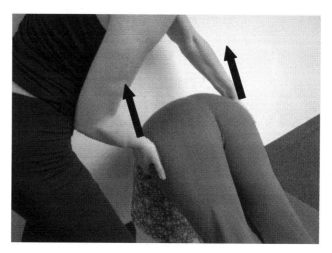

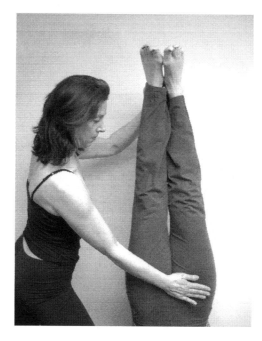

Assisting Steps for Headstand Pose (Supported)

Stand to one side of the person near their legs.

Check their head and arm placement in the base of the pose and offer verbal corrections (as in the top photo).

Place your hands in the thigh crease made by their bent legs with your fingers facing each other.

Give their hips a gentle lift as they float their hips up into headstand pose (as in the middle photo).

Once their legs are extended upward you can hold their ankles with one hand and give a lift.

Place your other arm in front of their hips (as in the bottom photo).

Now your can perform the fist squeeze as described later in this chapter.

Yoga Prop Suggestions

Have them perform this pose in front of a wall.

What You Might Say (to help the process)

"Push into your forearms," "Keep a firm hold on your head," "Press your shoulders down away from your ears," "Squeeze your inner thighs together."

> "I am 'taught' the assists in an 'ah-ha' moment when my own body is in a posture and something ignites. The assists grow from within me, so daily practice is my way to tending to that garden."
> —Kelly Smith, Yoga Teacher, Pilates Teacher

Inversions—Balancing with the Fist Squeeze

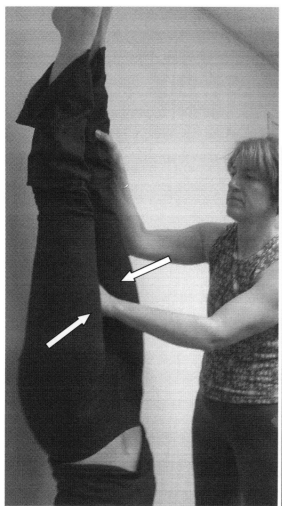 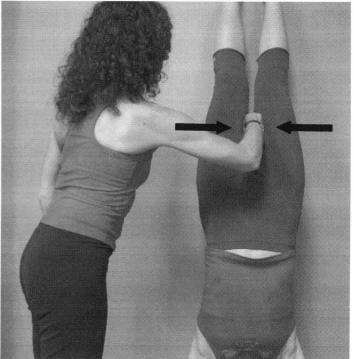

"Stop thinking about how you feel. Close your eyes and feel how you feel."
–Heidi Prewett, Devalila Yoga Teacher

Assisting Steps for the Fist Squeeze

NOTE: You can perform this adjustment on someone in an inversion such as handstand, forearm stand, or headstand.

Stand to one side or in front of the person near their legs.

Place one of your fists between their inner thighs (as in the right photo).

Instruct them to squeeze your fist with their legs and point their toes until they can balance on the own in the pose (without using the wall).

You can use your other hand to stabilize their legs (as in the left photo).

When they are steady in the pose, ask them to release your fist and let them balance on their own or with the help of the wall.

Yoga Prop Suggestions

Have them perform this pose in front of a wall.

What You Might Say (to help the process)

"Point your toes a lot," "Engage your abdominal muscles," "Squeeze your inner thighs together."

> "When you teach, just be yourself and share your experience. When you feel you don't want to teach, it's usually because you think you have to be someone other than who you are at the moment."
> —Stephanie Pappas, Devalila Yoga Teacher and Trainer

"Floating" into Headstand

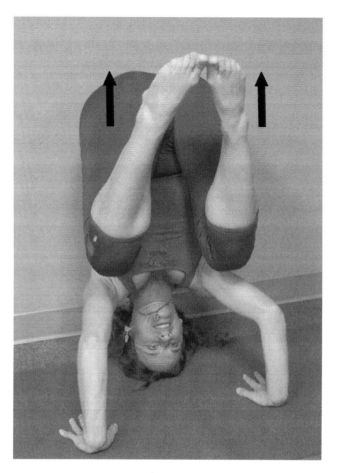

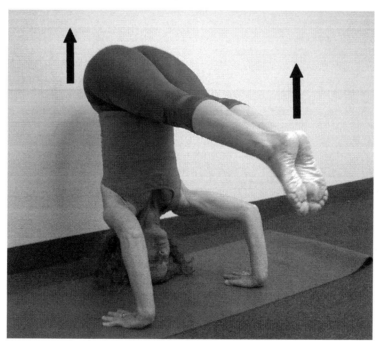

Tips on "Floating" into a Headstand Pose

Your hands and top of your head need to form a base like an equilateral triangle to create a solid foundation for your headstand.

If your head, neck, spine, pelvis and hips are in proper alignment in a headstand tripod preparation pose, then your legs may be able to "float"(as in the top photo) up into the full headstand pose.

Once you have established a solid base for your headstand, you can walk you feet inward toward your body until your hips stack over your shoulders.

Place your knees onto your triceps, firm your abdominal muscles, and bring your feet close to your hips.

At this point if your legs do not begin "floating" into the headstand, have the assistant check your alignment.

When your legs are straight it requires more abdominal strength to lift them into the headstand (as in the bottom photo). You may have to further develop your abdominal muscles to perform the straight leg variation.

Yoga Prop Suggestions

Perform this pose in front of a wall.

You can perform this pose outside on the grass on a flat surface.

Tips for Performing Inverted Postures

Inverted postures should be performed with utmost care and proper alignment.

Use blankets under your shoulders in shoulder stand, and plow pose. Make sure the blankets are FLAT!

Use a chair or the wall as support with plow or shoulder stand poses especially if you have excess body weight, or stiffness in neck and shoulders.

Use a flat blanket or yoga mat under your head for headstands.

Do not kick into a headstand. If you need to kick, then this indicates that you are improperly aligned, or have insufficient strength to perform the asana. Build up your abdominal muscles and keep stretching your neck and shoulders.

Get accustomed to headstand by practicing tri-pod headstand position without lifting your legs.

Do not "hang-out" in a headstand with your legs leaning against the wall. Touch the wall with your feet periodically to help with balance.

When the vertebrae align (because the body is strong and ready) in a headstand the feet will naturally "float" up. Trust the float principle!

Never perform a headstand on an unstable surface such as a bed, pillow or cushion!

Do not perform inverted poses immediately after eating. Wait 2-4 hours after eating before inverting or practicing yoga.

Beginners should hold the posture for a short time (under a minute) until there is no difficulty in maintaining the pose (1 minute or more). The duration can be increased gradually over time.

When using your forearms as the base of a headstand or forearm stand, make sure you start out with your elbows slightly closer than shoulder width apart. Elbows have a tendency to slide out during these poses and this can cause instability.

In a handstand pose, engage your legs, feet and inner thighs to lift upwards in the pose. Point your toes a lot.

Use the wall when first attempting headstand, handstand, forearm stand and scorpion poses.

Make sure to have a firm grip on your head in supported headstand pose. When the base of the pose is solid, the pose is steady!

Inverted poses should be followed by a resting pose until your heartbeat and breath return to normal. Child's pose is often suggested after a headstand. After resting in child's pose, return to an upright position like mountain pose (standing), or thunderbolt pose (kneeling).

Do not practice near objects, furniture, or anything that could hurt you if you fell.

I don't recommend closing your eyes during a headstand. Gaze to the floor in front of you, or at a point on the horizon.

If you fall out of an inversion remember to keep your body relaxed.

Use caution when practicing inversions if you have back or neck injuries, disc problems, or high blood pressure.

Some theories suggest avoiding inversions if you have detached retina, severe narrow angle glaucoma, osteoporosis, excess weight, you are pregnant, or you are menstruating.

If your eyes get bloodshot or you get broken blood vessels in your face after inverting, you may want to practice more gentle poses (downward dog, putting your legs up on a wall) until your body gets accustomed to inverting.

"Aside from the many practical benefits of physically assisting a student in the poses, a gentle touch can begin to break down physical and emotional barriers."
—Melissa Stern, Devalila Yoga Teacher

Sun Salutation Assisting Sequence

In this chapter I explain how you can dynamically assist someone as they move through the different postures of a traditional sun salutation sequence. If the person is a beginner, I suggest verbally instructing them in the poses as you are assisting them. If the person is already familiar with the sun salutation sequence, then you can simply let them move through the sequence at their own pace.

- Decide together ahead of time the approximate length of time, or number of breaths they will remain in each pose in the sequence.

- Remember to release the pressure when you sense they are about to move into another position.

- Remember to move out of their way as they transition from pose to pose.

- Anticipate and prepare your body position as they are transitioning from one pose to the next.

"When it feels like winter's dreary weight is separating you from where and who you would rather be, take a deep breath and realize that you will look back on this time remembering that you were actually running through summer's open pastures."
–Marc Savoie, Yoga Student

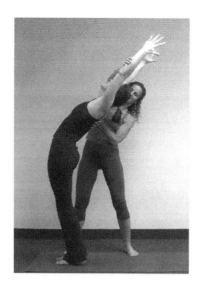

Position 1: *Arching Mountain*

Stand to the person's side and use one of you hands to lift their upper back between the shoulder blades. Use your other hand to press both their forearms backward. Release and let them move into the next position —forward fold.

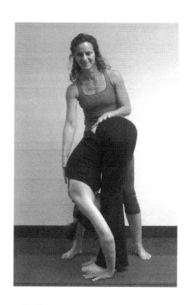

Position 2: *Forward Fold*

Stand at the same side and move your hand (from their shoulder blades) down to rest on their sacrum as they fold forward. Use your other hand to press down on their back to help them stretch into the forward fold. Release and let them move into the next position—lunge.

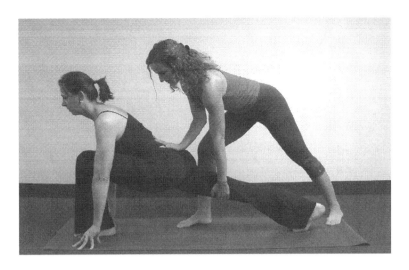

Position 3: High Lunge (right leg back)

Position yourself in a low lunge position so that you can reach their body (you can also straddle their back leg). Simultaneously, press down in the center of their sacrum with one hand (your fingers are facing up), and lift their leg up with your other hand. Find a balance between pushing down on the sacrum and lifting up on the back leg. Release and let them move into the next position—high plank.

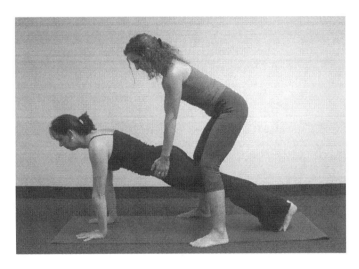

Position 4: High Plank

Straddle their legs around the thigh area. Lift their hips up or down in alignment with their legs and torso. Hold their hips up as they lower their body into the next pose—Caterpillar.

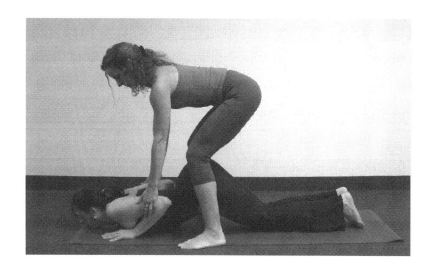

Position 5: Caterpillar
Stand in a deep squat position over their hips and press their elbows toward their body. Release and let them move into the next position—cobra.

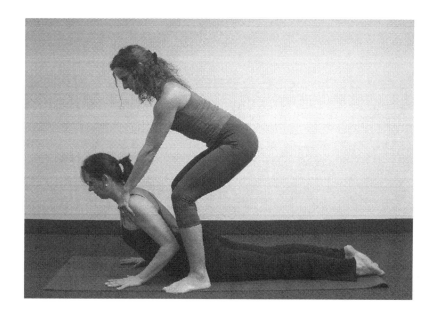

Position 6: Cobra
Move your hands onto the fronts of their shoulders and lift their body up. Release and let them move into the next position—downward dog.

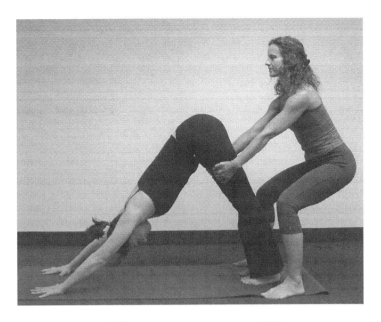

Position 7: Downward Dog

Step backward and place your feet outside their feet as they press their hips up. Hold their upper thighs and sink your weight backward into a deep squat. Release and let them move into the next position—lunge.

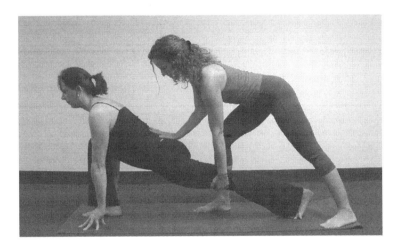

Position 8: High Lunge (right leg forward)

Step into a low lunge position so that you can reach their body (you can also straddle their back leg). Simultaneously, press down in the center of their sacrum with one hand (your fingers facing up), and lift their leg up with your other hand. Find a balance between pushing down on the sacrum and lifting up on the back leg. Release and let them move into the next position—forward fold.

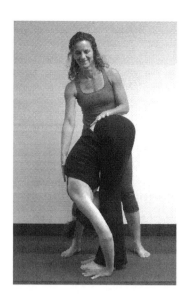

Position 9: Forward Fold

Stand to one side of the person and place your hand on their sacrum. Use your other hand to press down on their back to help them stretch deeper into the forward fold. Release and let them move into the next position—arching mountain.

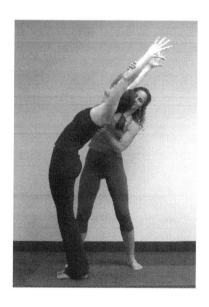

Position 10: Arching Mountain

Lift between their shoulder blades with your closest hand. Use your other arm to press both their extended arms backward. Release and let them move into a normal standing position.

Section III

Candid Replies to Questions

You Were Hesitant to Ask

Replies to Questions from Yoga Teachers

In this section I would like to reflect upon some questions and concerns raised by yoga teachers. My hope is that after reading this section you will feel a greater sense self-acceptance in regard to your unique experiences as a yoga teacher.

My responses in this section are based on 14 years of experience practicing and teaching yoga, and also on thousands of personal conversations and intimate discussions with hundreds of yoga teachers from all styles, backgrounds, and levels of experience.

Sometimes I feel internal conflict. I teach all this spiritual stuff and appear so centered in class, but when I am alone I sometimes feel anxious, depressed, unhappy, or sad. Should I be teaching yoga?

> Of course, you can still teach yoga. To me, yoga practice includes all that happens in life—including intense emotions. It seems to me that we find our inner wisdom through all of these experiences—pleasant or unpleasant. When I experience intense emotions, I work with them as I would work with a yoga posture.
>
> I have often heard this question, and I wonder where teachers and students get such unrealistic, super human notions about yoga teachers. In my experience, the challenges and painful times in life make us more compassionate, authentic, and aware of our own habit patterns.
>
> Maybe you can teach your class from a space of greater honesty and authenticity. Weave your personal life experiences into the class, and encourage your students to embrace the totality of who they are. Somewhere along the way, maybe you bought into someone else's ideas about what it means to be a yoga teacher. Reflect upon what spirituality means to you at this time in your life.

I feel nervous before teaching and sometimes during the class. Is this normal? Is there anything I can do? Why do I feel this way?

In my experience, I have noticed different causes behind the feeling of nervousness in myself when teaching. I hope you will be able to identify with something that I am about to write, and that what I share will ease the burden you may feel.

There is a type of nervousness that comes when you are a new teacher and you are not that confident. This is bound to happen, but with more experience and practice it will diminish. Remember that you can use the breathing practices to relax and center yourself. Usually, once you start doing some postures the nervous feelings fade.

There is also the kind of nervousness that comes when you are stepping into unknown territory and sharing deeper parts of yourself with groups of people. I think this is actually a good sign—a sign that you have expressed yourself fully, openly, and with less censorship. When I really share myself and express myself in class, afterwards I sometimes feel vulnerable and uncomfortable.

There is another kind of nervousness that is more like excitement or exhilaration that you may experience while teaching. It is natural to feel this way when you love what you are doing, and truly feel the joy of sharing it. Most of the time your students really appreciate you and you can feel this positive energy in your body.

The last type of nervousness I will mention can manifest when we feel doubtful, fearful, or low in our self-esteem. There are certain times in life when we feel this way. It is just part of the journey, but it is often very uncomfortable. Do the best you can, and remember that most people have these feelings. Life is a mystery and you can experience a full spectrum of feelings during your journey here.

What do I do when I don't feel like teaching, but have made a commitment to teach?

This is a great question and so many teachers have shared this question with me.

Unless I am really sick, or have travel problems, I teach class anyway, despite my feelings. I know that feelings just keep changing and changing. Almost always, I feel better after I have taught a class. It is a good way to get out of our own self-absorbed state.

Just keep showing up for your commitments, change them when you are ready, and do so in a way that also honors all the people involved. There were a few times when I felt ready to leave a particular class or venue; so I fulfilled my commitment, and then stopped teaching the class.

The more interesting part of this situation is that you can go deeper into what you are feeling and what's behind not feeling like teaching. Pay closer attention to the feelings and senses you are having in your body. While feeling the feelings, listen inwardly to any thoughts that come to your mind. You may get some new insights about your current life situation.

There are many reasons for not wanting to teach:

Sometimes we do not feel physically well.
We may be dealing with overwhelming emotional distress.
We may have temporarily lost our enthusiasm for teaching.
There may be phases when we feel inadequate.
We might not be receiving adequate compensation for our time.
We may be going through a period of questioning our beliefs and practices.
We may feel that it is time to move on from the particular group or venue.
We may not like the environment in which we are teaching.

All of these experiences are valid and worth exploring.

Another more subtle reason for not wanting to teach could be that you feel you aren't quite being yourself. Once I had an experience teaching yoga at a spa in a tourist environment. The owner sometimes came to my classes, and at times wanted me to intentionally make the people sweat. This attitude was not in harmony with mine, so I eventually stopped teaching yoga at this place. You have to be true to yourself and teach what is real for you. Even if no one else is teaching how you teach, you have to take a risk and be yourself. It may not be easy for you, but it is an opportunity to express yourself completely.

What do I do when I feel strong dislike for a student?

Does the student do something that feels dishonoring to you? Have you not spoken your true feelings or needs to them? Have you lost touch with your values or boundaries in some way? Is it possible to have a personal talk with this person, or write to them about what you are feeling without placing blame or guilt?

I find that students can awaken personal issues that we have within ourselves—they can push our buttons so to speak. You may find it valuable to work with an experienced therapist. It is important to deal with the feelings that arise from being with your students. I am not saying it is easy to take responsibility for your feelings, but it seems to be the healthiest thing to do. Remember that the student may be reflecting some aspect of the "shadow" side of your personality. I highly recommend the book, "The Dark Side of the Light Chasers," by Debbie Ford, if you would like to explore this concept further.

What can I do when I am sexually attracted to a student?

You can let the feelings pass by, and focus your attention back on the class. If the feelings are mutual between you and the student, then it may be appropriate to have an honest conversation about it and together decide your course of action. You may decide to terminate your professional relationship and pursue the personal relationship. In my experience, it's healthier to focus on one or the other, but not both at the same time. Each individual must take personal responsibility for their choices and decisions.

What should I do if I have a physical problem while teaching class and I can't continue the class?

I would explain to the class what is happening (with as many or as few details as is comfortable for you). I would also refund their money, or give them credit toward a future class.

I have read in yogic texts and from certain teachers that a yoga teacher should be a vegetarian and live certain principles of a yogic life style. I don't feel I am living up to these standards. Should I be teaching yoga?

Your lifestyle is a personal decision which is based on many factors. I don't feel a yoga teacher must to be a vegetarian in order to teach. I invite you to question everything you hear and read. Learn to listen to your inner wisdom and make choices based on your deepest values. You may go through certain phases in your life. Keep noticing how you feel and what your body is requesting of you.

Sometimes I can't do my own yoga practice or meditate. Does this mean I shouldn't be a teacher?

You are a teacher. Find a balance between freedom and discipline that feels honoring to you. Your practice may go through different phases. I have been through years of intense practice, and times of none. I used to beat myself up for the times of not practicing. Now I recognize that we all express our spirituality in different ways at different times. What works for you? Are you practicing in a way that suits your style? Are you just following someone else's plan? Find your own unique way to practice. Listen and let it flow. Don't give up on yourself or the practice, and let go of the guilt as much as possible.

I have a student that appears to be viewing my body sexually during class and I feel uncomfortable. What can I do?

I would address that person directly and immediately, face to face. Select your words carefully so that they won't feel you are blaming them. Remember that there is the possibility that you are projecting on them. If you still do not feel comfortable with their behavior after the conversation, you could politely ask them to leave the class.

What do I do if I have a student that makes too much noise or is disruptive in my class?

If the student is making noises as a form of emotional release, then I would allow them to continue making these sounds. If other class members are bothered by these sounds then they have to handle it in their own way. You can have an open discussion in class.

There are some situations where the disruption is physical in nature and could cause harm to other students. In this case, I would immediately speak to the student. If a student is making too many side comments or jokes, you may want to speak to them after class and suggest that they do this outside of class.

What can I do when a student won't stop performing poses in an unsafe way, and they won't follow my instructions?

If they won't stop or change their unsafe behavior after you have repeatedly attempted to correct them, then you should leave them alone and focus on other students. If they are doing something that puts another student in danger, then you should firmly ask them to stop or leave the class. Ultimately they are responsible for themselves. Have them sign a release form stating that you are not responsible for any injuries occurring in class.

I don't feel enthusiastic about teaching anymore. Should I quit? What can I do?

This can happen. You can take a break from teaching. You can do a workshop in something that inspires you (yoga or another subject). Maybe you are just teaching too much, or in places that don't like. Maybe you need to change your schedule. It is important to explore what you are experiencing and make some changes.

There are times when yoga teachers, like any other professional, want to change their job. Stay open to the changes.

What can I do if a student is doing their own practice during class and won't listen to any of my instructions?

This can be really distracting to the teacher and the other students! I would ask them to move to the rear of the room the next time they come to class.

If they won't listen to your instructions at all, it's a wonder that they are even in class. Maybe it is their ego or they are just showing off. You can refer them to another style of yoga class that is self-led and may suit them better. If you feel they are just trying to get your attention, offer them a private session.

I feel it is healthy for students to listen to their bodies and make adjustments and variations in their practice. I encourage freedom and individuality in my classes.

What can I do if a student talks too much after class and I find myself spending more time than I would like with them?

Get clearer on your personal boundaries. Be attentive, but don't get pulled into their neediness. Politely tell them that you would like to share with them, but another time would be better for you. Request that they call you at a specific time, or communicate with you via email. You can refer them to a therapist or to another health care specialist if their concerns or questions are out of your field of experience.

I am a female teacher. What do I say if a female student invites me out after class and wants to be friends with me?

In the field of yoga I have not read any specific rules prohibiting friendships between teachers and students. Other professions have strict codes of conduct in this regard.

In my opinion, when the feeling is mutual and both people want to cultivate a friendship, then it can be pursued. Together, decide on a protocol for your relationship. Make sure you are both clear and understand what your roles are in the classroom.

Personally, I can report that some of my current best friends are previous yoga students. I have not had a bad experience cultivating a same sex friendship.

What can I do if a student of the opposite sex asks me out for a date, or expresses interest in starting a relationship with me?

This is tricky. Be honest, but kind to the person. If the feeling is mutual, you both have to decide what you want to do. I would choose between the teacher-student relationship or the courtship. In my experience, it works better if it is one or the other. Just remember that there could be an imbalance of power in the future relationship because you were in the teacher's role when you met.

When I substitute for other teachers I experience some negative energy from some of the students in their class. What can I do?

This can be uncomfortable. Do the best you can, be yourself, and teach in your own style. They are just accustomed to their own favorite teacher, and they are probably disappointed that he or she is not there for class. Do your job and focus your attention on the students who are more open and receptive. The negative vibes usually fade during the class as they focus on their yoga practice. If possible, don't take it too personally.

When other yoga teachers come to my class I feel they are judging me, and checking me out. I feel uncomfortable and self-conscious when this happens. What can I do?

Be friendly to them, be yourself, and just teach your class as you would normally teach it. If they are feeling competitive, then it is their issue to handle. If you are feeling competitive or doubtful about yourself, then it is your issue to explore.

I feel awkward when a certain friends or family members come to my yoga class. What can I do?

It can be awkward at first when someone we know from another part of our life sees us in a different light, or in a different role. In this situation, our own personal history is mixing with our professional life. In my experience it works best if the both of you can be in class in professional manner and mentally put aside the personal aspects of the relationship. Is their behavior in class inappropriate or disrespectful to you as a teacher? Maybe you need to talk with them about it.

At times I have gas pains, or have to release gas while teaching. It is uncomfortable and distracting. What can I do to prevent or deal with this?

Don't eat too much or too soon before class. Examine your diet with a qualified Ayurvedic practitioner or nutrition specialist. Use the bathroom before you teach class, and go out for a bathroom break if you really need it. Otherwise, attempt to let it out silently, or maybe open the windows and light incense!

When a student regularly or occasionally farts in class and other people in the class laugh, should I address it or just ignore it?

It depends on the situation and the atmosphere in your class. Usually I just ignore it and focus on what we are doing in class. There have been a few occasions where I have made appropriate comments.

What if I find it hard to teach when I am menstruating? I feel like I would rather just be alone or rest.

This is a common experience with female teachers I know. Sometimes we have to just get a substitute to teach for us. Sometimes we can let the class flow from the state we are in. Maybe at this time of the month you can allow your class to have a different tone then it usually does (perhaps a more inward focus, or a slower pace).

I have some students that seem disinterested in what I have to say and look all around the room when I am talking. I find this uncomfortable, is there anything I can do?

Focus on the students that look interested. If you focus on the disinterested students, your energy may be affected. If this behavior happens on a regular basis, I would have a private talk with them to find out what they are experiencing. Avoid using language that could suggest that you are blaming or judging them.

When I have been emotionally unstable some people have said, "You are a yoga teacher, shouldn't you be beyond that already?" I feel uncomfortable, and it seems as if they are projecting an image on me. How should I respond?

Avoid getting defensive and invite them into a conversation about it. You could ask them some questions about how they view yoga teachers, or what they have heard. Maybe they think yoga teachers are somehow immune to human suffering. Maybe they expect the yoga practices to stop emotions. It could be an interesting discussion.

Hopefully, by the time the conversation is over, they will have a better understanding. You could share with them that you are in the process of deepening your understanding of life, and that you also go through ups and downs. You could also share how yoga has helped you deal with the challenges. Remind them that you are human.

I noticed a student crying during class. Should I talk to them, comfort them, or just let them be?

That depends on the student, the class, your relationship, and the type of crying. You may want to check in with them after class. If they are crying intensely, I would approach them and ask if I can help in some way. In certain cases just the simplest act of just bringing them a tissue is enough to acknowledge their tears. I have had students ask me after class if this is normal. I always tell them that it is normal and healthy to cry.

If I can't do a certain posture, should I teach it anyway?

You can teach a posture to the best of your ability even if you can't perform it in its full expression. You can use props to help you demonstrate. If you can step someone else through the posture safely, then it is probably alright to teach it. If you feel uncomfortable with the pose and you can't demonstrate it or explain it well, then I don't recommend teaching it.

Replies to Questions from Yoga Students

We can experience so many different types of thoughts and feelings while we are in a yoga class, or practicing on our own. There are times when our experiences can raise big or small questions in our minds. Sometimes insights come from our own direct life experience, and sometimes they can come from hearing about the experiences of others. In this section I hope that my comments may provide some insight into questions you may have. I aspire to lighten your load, heighten your awareness, and provoke more questions in you.

Sometimes I feel self-conscious in yoga class. Is this normal?

I think it's normal. Be patient with yourself. I know very few people who haven't felt self-conscious at one time or another. I suggest that you go a little deeper into the sensations that accompany the self-consciousness. What is going on in your mind? I have had this experience at times and found that the feelings dissolved over time as I became more comfortable with myself, the yoga practice, and the teacher.

I feel that I am infatuated, and maybe even in love with my teacher. Should I approach him/her? What should I do with these feelings?

I think it is common to feel loving feelings toward someone who is a positive force in your life, cares for you, and shows an interest in your greater well-being. It is good to communicate your feelings if you feel the need, and at the same time keep the reality of the situation in mind. I think it is important stay unattached to the results of your communication with the teacher. Remember to respect the professional boundaries of the teacher.

Even though I know yoga is not about competition I find myself looking at other students and comparing myself. I don't want to do this, but it happens anyway. Do you have any suggestions?

This is a very honest question. I have noticed many students doing this in class. I know that most all of us have felt competitive in life at one time or another. Well, at least you are aware of it! So when you catch yourself doing it, just bring your focus once again to your body, your breath, or the feelings behind your impulse to be competitive. It is all part of the process of yoga. We are becoming more aware of our habits, tendencies and mental patterns. Certain mind-body types have this tendency more than others. If you are curious, read more about the "pitta" body type in Ayurveda.

Sometimes I feel like the teacher is reading my mind and making comments directly to me. I am imagining things?

On one level we are all connected, and your time in a yoga class can be a very personal and unique experience. I think it is normal for the teacher to be aware of what is happening with you and the other students. It may be that many people in the class are having a similar experience and the teacher is picking up on it. Sometimes your teacher will be more in tune than other times. You can accept the comments as a gift and appreciate the mystery of the experience, but I wouldn't take it too personally.

Once in a while I feel angry with the teacher for making us do certain things in class. Why?

There are different reasons why you may feel angry: the teacher may be over-zealous or lack empathy, you may be pushing yourself too hard, you may be physically over-heated, you may be angry at something else, or you may be picking up on someone else's anger.

In the first case, the teacher may be pushing you too hard in class, or not instructing to your level of ability. Once a student told me that they felt angry because a teacher asked the class to perform headstands, but did not offer any instruction for how to build into a headstand for the students who were unfamiliar with the techniques. If this is the case, I would suggest speaking to the teacher after class and offer your feedback.

You may feel angry because you are not honoring your body and resting when you need to if the class is getting too challenging. Listen to your own needs and body signals.

If you have the type of body that gets over-heated easily and the room or climate is too hot, you may find yourself feeling irritated. I definitely have experienced this! Certain types of vigorous hot yoga classes may not be good for your body type. For more information on this, read about Ayurveda and the pitta body type according to Ayurveda.

I want the teacher to notice me when I do a pose well. Is this my ego?

Yes and no. I think we learn to look for outside approval when we are young. We want to be good students and children. We look to others for validation and feedback. Wanting feedback for what we are doing is a natural thing. We are dynamic beings and get information about ourselves from the world around us. Maybe a private yoga session with the teacher would help clarify any doubts you have about the postures.

Also, you could become more aware the motives behind your desire. Why do you want the teacher to notice you in a pose? Do you have this tendency in other aspects of your life as well? Can you bring your attention back to yourself when you catch it happening? It is all good juicy stuff to use for increased self-awareness and empathy toward others who may be feeling the same way.

I notice sexual feelings arising in my body during class. Is this from the postures?

It is possible. I have found that the postures definitely stimulate our bodies physically and energetically in many ways. Maybe you were feeling sexual before class and just became more aware of it? Sexuality is part of our human nature. Feelings can arise anywhere, anytime.

Notice if you are intentionally provoking or seeking some experience from class. Be honest with yourself.

There are certain people in class that repel me and I don't want to be next to them in class. Is it okay for me to move my mat?

Do what feels right to you about your placement in class, and also notice if you are projecting your judgments onto the person. I think it is natural to be attracted to some people and repelled by others in life. Is there something you can learn about yourself from the experience? How are you like them? Have you ever been like them? You never know…they could end up being your best friend.

I sometimes have problems with gas when I do yoga. Do you have any advice?

Most books and professionals suggest refraining from yoga practice 2-4 hours after eating. If you are practicing yoga soon after eating you may be upsetting your digestive system.

Some of the postures put pressure on the colon and small intestines, and help to relieve excess gas. This is great for you, but not so great for your classmates! There always seems to be that moment of uncertainty with accidental farting. We wonder if we should excuse ourselves, or act as if it didn't happen. If you are in a yoga class, I think it's probably best to ignore it and keep practicing.

You may also want to look more closely at your diet, and investigate food allergies/food sensitivities you may have. It may be time for some type of digestive cleansing regime.

I have a lot of nasal discharge during breathing practices. Is this common?

Certain vigorous pranayama practices like bhastrika or kapalabhati can release mucous from your sinuses. Bring tissues with you to class. If it needs to flow, then let it flow!

I sometimes cry during or after class. Do other people experience this? I thought yoga was supposed to make you feel good and happy!

To me, the yoga practice is about feeling more, not less. Maybe you just didn't have time to notice the feelings before. I have experienced crying in class and after class, and so have many other teachers and students that I know. We are becoming more aware of our body, thoughts, and feelings. Sometimes we cry because we are touched by something said or felt in class, and sometimes we are just feeling sad.

Sometimes I feel like modifying a posture or doing a different posture than the teacher is suggesting. Is this okay?

In some styles of yoga this is okay, and in some it is not. In my classes, I encourage the students to listen to their own body wisdom and modify the posture if necessary. If you are performing lots of postures that are different from what the teaching is instructing, then I would suggest going to the back of the room so that your actions don't disturb the teacher or the other students.

I find myself comparing myself to the teacher and sometimes I feel inadequate and jealous. How can I get over this?

It is natural to respect and admire your teacher. If these feelings are coming up, I suggest putting the focus back on yourself, your uniqueness, and your good qualities. I have compared myself to the teacher at times when I doubted myself. Investigate what else you want to do in your life and how to develop or express your creative talents.

Is it okay to leave during a class if you really find you don't want to be there?

Yes, I think so. I have done that a few times. It may mess with the teacher's mind, but they will handle it. If you have a long term relationship with the teacher, you may want to call them and share your experience.

I really appreciate my teacher and would like to give a gift. Is this appropriate?

I think it is appropriate if there are no hidden motives behind your gift, and if you are not attached to any results of giving the gift. When my students have given me gifts from a sincere place, I was able to openly receive them.

I find it hard to focus when I practice yoga on my own. Is this common? What can help me practice alone?

This is such a common question! I think it's partially because the yoga practice is unfamiliar to us at the beginning and it naturally takes us awhile to cultivate new habits and hobbies in life. Also, if you are unfamiliar with spending time alone, then it may be even more challenging. If you are practicing at home, create or find a space with few distractions. I find it easier to practice when I am outside in a natural setting. Try playing some music and dance freely before doing the more formal practices.

Give yourself small, manageable goals in the beginning. For example, agree to just practice one or two postures per day and see what happens from there.

I can't meditate. My mind never shuts up. What am I doing wrong?

It's not wrong to have thoughts, is it? In meditation we become even more aware of our thoughts as a part of the process of self-inquiry. Part of the mind's nature is to contemplate, visualize, reflect and analyze. Sometimes the thinking process is interesting and satisfying. Sure, when our mental chatter spins out of control, and we are focusing on negative thoughts, it can be quite unpleasant and even stressful. Nonetheless, it is still a part of the process. Meditation is awareness of all and everything we do—including thinking. Don't make an enemy of your mind. It is part of you. Become aware of the thoughts and be gentle on your mind.

When the teacher comes over to assist me I feel distracted, singled-out, and I can't relax. Do you have any suggestions help me get the most out of the personal attention I am getting?

Focus on your breath. Focus on what you are feeling. Let go and let them move you. Over time you will get used to the attention and not take it so personally.

If I smoke, drink and eat meat does this mean that I am a bad yoga practitioner, or shouldn't practice yoga?

In my opinion, you are not a bad yoga practitioner, and by all means keep practicing if you enjoy the practice. How you live and what you do is personal. If you don't like doing these things and you are harming yourself, then work at changing your behavior. All experiences are part of life. Ask for help when you need it.

There is another student in the class that breathes heavily and makes emotional noises which distract me. What should I do?

You could pick a spot farthest spot away from that person. Often the teacher can't do anything about it because every student has a right to be there and express themselves freely. You could also pick a spot right next to the person and work with the situation as a means of cultivating patience, acceptance and concentration!

Sometimes I feel dizzy when I get up from a pose. Is there something wrong with me?

This could be a result of a rapid change in blood pressure when you get up. Maybe you didn't eat enough that day. When your head is below your body for period of time in a pose, stand up very slowly and gradually.

I feel guilty if I don't practice regularly. Do you have any comments?

I love this question. I have felt this too! Ultimately, discipline is subjective and personal. Set manageable goals for yourself and relax when you don't reach them. Maybe you have your expectations set too high.

Remember, there is no one watching. Whose rules are you trying to follow? You will probably enjoy the practice and do it more often if you let go of what you think you "should" be doing, and follow your inner wisdom.

I feel ashamed of my body and have a negative self-image. Will this improve by practicing yoga?

I have observed that yoga practices improve people's self-image, but I can't say for sure that they will for you. I certainly don't think practicing yoga can hurt your self-image. You may want to investigate the thought patterns and mental conditioning you have regarding your body and self-image. Meditation is a great way to catch those thoughts in action. Maybe you can seek out an experienced counselor or therapist with experience in this area.

About the Author

Stephanie (a.k.a. Stefani) Ann Pappas has been practicing and teaching yoga since 1992, and is an Experienced Registered Yoga Teacher (ERYT) at the 500 hour level with Yoga Alliance. Stephanie began directing yoga teacher trainings in 1999. In 2002, she founded the Devalila Yoga Teacher Training program, a registered 200 hour level training with Yoga Alliance, and has certified over 100 teachers since 1999. She is also a massage therapist, interfaith minister, ESL teacher, and aspiring web designer.

Stephanie has practiced different forms of movement throughout of her life including gymnastics, running, hiking, mountain biking, and martial arts. Her current focus is yoga and dance. She holds regular yoga classes, yoga teacher trainings, and belly dance classes for women in the U.S.A in New Jersey, and in Mexico. Stephanie offers yoga books and belly dance practice DVDs for sale on her websites: www.devalilayoga.com and www.yogapostureadjustments.com

She continues to wonder about life, love, and relationships.

Stephanie is available for classes, workshops, and seminars worldwide.

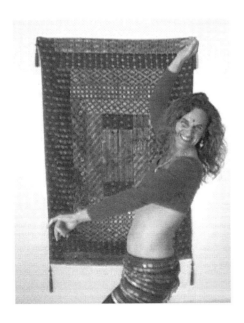 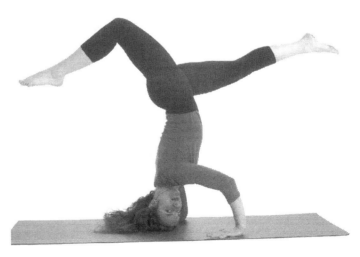

ISBN 141205162-2

Made in the USA
Lexington, KY
06 August 2013